Occupational Therapy
and Dementia

D1333899

of related interest

Why Dementia Makes Communication Difficult
A Guide to Better Outcomes
Alison Wray
ISBN 978 1 78775 606 9
eISBN 978 1 78775 607 6

A Clinician's Guide to Non-Pharmacological Dementia Therapies
Daniel Nightingale
ISBN 978 1 78592 595 5
eISBN 978 1 78592 602 0

CLEAR Dementia Care©
A Model to Assess and Address Unmet Needs
Dr Frances Duffy
ISBN 978 1 78592 276 3
eISBN 978 1 78775 462 1

The Essential Guide for Newly Qualified Occupational Therapists
Transition to Practice
Edited by Ruth Parker and Julia Badger
ISBN 978 1 78592 268 8
eISBN 978 1 78450 558 5

OCCUPATIONAL THERAPY and DEMENTIA

Promoting Inclusion, Rights and Opportunities for People Living with Dementia

EDITED BY

Fiona Maclean, Alison Warren, Elaine Hunter and Lyn Westcott

Forewords by Scottish Dementia Working Group, including Wendy Rankin, and Professor Clare Hocking

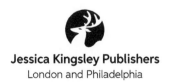

Jessica Kingsley Publishers
London and Philadelphia

First published in Great Britain in 2023 by Jessica Kingsley Publishers
An imprint of Hodder & Stoughton Ltd
An Hachette UK Company

1

Copyright © Jessica Kingsley Publishers 2023

The right of Fiona Maclean, Alison Warren, Elaine Hunter & Lyn Westcott
to be identified as the Author of the Work has been asserted by them in
accordance with the Copyright, Designs and Patents Act 1988.

Foreword © Wendy Rankin 2023
Foreword © Professor Clare Hocking 2023

A CIP catalogue record for this title is available from the
British Library and the Library of Congress

ISBN 978 1 83997 062 7
eISBN 978 1 83997 061 0

Printed and bound by CPI Group (UK) Ltd, Croydon, CR0 4YY

Jessica Kingsley Publishers' policy is to use papers that are natural, renewable
and recyclable products and made from wood grown in sustainable
forests. The logging and manufacturing processes are expected to conform
to the environmental regulations of the country of origin.

Jessica Kingsley Publishers
Carmelite House
50 Victoria Embankment
London EC4Y 0DZ

www.jkp.com

For Bruce and Dorothy, with thanks to Neil, Struan, and Ellen. (FM)

To my parents who encouraged me to join a truly inspiring profession, with thanks to Mandy and Steve. (AW)

For Tom and June, with thanks to Iain, Ewan, and Craig. (EH)

Contents

Section 3: Occupation

Foreword

As members of the Scottish Dementia Working Group (SDWG), we all have different interests. Some of us like to sing, to play bowls, to go to the gym, or to continue to enjoy socializing with friends and family. If we were to meet in person, we would be like you, the reader of this book. We would be able to find points of interest in common and to enjoy each other's company – the only difference being that we have a diagnosis of dementia, and you do not.

Often, our experience has been that once you or others hear we have a diagnosis of dementia, it can change how you see us, how you understand us, and how you may respond towards us. A diagnosis of dementia can become a stigma – a horrible word – which can mean our potential to continue to live positive lives for longer is diminished.

As a result, the SDWG is a national member-led campaigning and awareness-raising group, for people living with a diagnosis of dementia in Scotland. To be a member of our group you must have a diagnosis of dementia and hold a commitment towards the promotion of human rights for all those living with dementia.

This means we try to raise awareness of what people living with dementia can continue to do and achieve, amongst health, social care and related professions, as well as the wider public. Over recent years this has led us to work in partnership with occupational therapy students and graduates.

Through various projects, we have shared with them our experiences and stories of what it is to live with a diagnosis of dementia. In so doing, we think this is helping to change how occupational therapy students and graduates think – to value and see the person living with dementia, not the diagnosis; to work in partnership with those living with dementia, where we can learn new skills together, which build on abilities, as opposed to disability; and to treat the person with dementia with dignity and respect. There is still a person there.

We have enjoyed working with occupational therapy students and graduates, and as a result, we wanted to support and contribute to this book. We see it as an opportunity to build more knowledge and understanding of dementia. In working with a range of allied health professionals, including occupational therapists, we hope this book will offer you a broader understanding of dementia. There is a lot of good work going on, and we want you to know about it.

More importantly, as the future of your profession, we hope you will be inspired to continue to progress the contribution of occupational therapy to the lives of those living with dementia. And in so doing, to highlight that people living with dementia can continue to contribute to a variety of different activities, in different ways. You are the future, and together we can make a positive difference to our future.

Scottish Dementia Working Group (SDWG), including
Wendy Rankin, Active Voice Lead (SDWG)

Foreword

In my first year as a practising occupational therapist in the 1980s, I met an older woman diagnosed with Alzheimer's disease. I have long since forgotten her name, but I'll call her Ethel, an old-fashioned English name that means 'noble'. Ethel had been admitted to a respite bed in a 'back' ward of a public hospital in Christchurch, New Zealand, where people with severe health conditions who required 'heavy nursing care' lived out their days. Such wards typically had a few short-stay beds to admit people from the community for a couple of weeks of rehabilitation and to give their carers a break. What I do vividly remember is how Ethel fluctuated between a contented state of confusion, when she was carried along by whatever was happening in the ward, and acute anxiety. At those times, she clearly understood that she was losing her grasp on who she was, where she was, and the life she had led. The inevitable loss of self was a terrifying prospect, and Ethel's best hope, as I understood it then, was to sink into a more peaceful state of permanent not knowing.

Looking back, several aspects of this story are astonishing. For instance, it is surprising that, in my early twenties, I had never interacted with someone with dementia in my family or community settings. Thus, I could see Ethel's distress, but had no experience to draw from to approach, calm or interact with her. Projections about the rapid increase in rates of dementia amongst older adults, as a direct consequence of population ageing (WHO 2021a), suggest this lack of exposure will not be the norm for young people in the future. Also astonishing is the pervading sense of hopelessness that surrounded Ethel. Her fate was sealed – a steady decline into incapacity and loss of personhood – with attention turning to how her husband might be supported in the taxing job of providing 24-hour care. A diagnosis of dementia was a cruel fate, not least because of the stigma (and self-stigma) it attracted and the future it invoked: loss of social graces, institutionalization and premature death. Most terrifying, as a recent graduate, I had no idea what occupational therapy might offer. Maybe I missed that lecture. But what could possibly make a difference when she was deposited in an unfamiliar environment and had no access to her everyday life, routines, interests, skills, motivations or memories? Forty years later, Ethel has certainly passed away. I do not recall doing anything that made a material difference to her situation; I hope she forgave me.

The intervening 40 years have not produced the cure many hoped for, nor, to my knowledge, decreased the rates of early onset dementia. There is, however, increasing evidence from research about the capabilities and rights of people with dementia and deep attitudinal change towards dementia. Occupational therapy has been instrumental in that shift. When I first partnered with Dr Grace O'Sullivan in the early 2000s to improve the lives of people with dementia, the landscape was bleak. As Morris Friedell (2003), a speaker at an Alzheimer's Association conference in the USA, asserted, the biomedical focus on the debilitating symptoms of dementia painted a picture of a catastrophic illness. As a person diagnosed with Alzheimer's disease, Friedell was at liberty to use such dramatic language. The medical focus on charting the negative outcomes and caregiver burden perpetuated fear, patronizing attitudes and stigma (O'Sullivan, Hocking and Spence 2014b). At the time, little practical and research attention was being given to living with dementia, let alone *living well* with dementia. Perhaps most damaging was that, in the absence of hope, people receiving a diagnosis of dementia responded to the negative stereotyping. They feared the worst, mourned their losses, hid their condition, and prematurely withdrew from occupations at home, at work and in their communities, thus setting in motion a cycle of excess disability. In the face of systemic failure to understand the needs and capabilities of people with dementia, it was unimaginable that dementia was 'not necessarily something to be afraid of' (O'Sullivan *et al.* 2014b, p.494).

Occupational therapy's contribution to turning that situation around rests on the profession's core belief that occupations give purpose, meaning, identity, opportunities for enjoyment and satisfaction; in short, they make life worth living and promote health. Even in the advanced stages of dementia, there is nothing to suggest that people have a diminished need for occupation. Indeed, the need to actively engage may be greater, given that participation in occupation engages the brain. For all these reasons, occupational therapists fully appreciate that one of the most debilitating outcomes of dementia, with profound consequences for the person, is the loss of occupation (Taylor 2007). Understanding this makes clear where our responsibilities lie. We must seek occupational justice for people with dementia (O'Sullivan and Hocking 2013). This means both generating and applying knowledge that will pave the way to maintenance of functional abilities and living a rich life. More than that, we must become guardians of a hopeful discourse of enablement, disseminators of everyday actions that support inclusion, and champions of knowledge that breaks down socially constructed prejudices. Through these actions, as we educate individuals and influence societal attitudes, we can challenge the demoralizing ways people with dementia have been treated by family, friends, colleagues, shop assistants, banking staff – indeed, everyone, particularly health professionals, with whom they come into contact (O'Sullivan, Hocking and Spence 2014a).

Occupational Therapy and Dementia: Promoting Inclusion, Rights and Opportunities for People Living with Dementia both reflects and promotes that shift in perspective. My confidence in making that assertion comes first from inclusion of the voices of people with dementia. Whatever else changes, it is not enough until people with dementia are active in the conversation and respected as informants, research partners and citizens, with full rights to inclusion. The concept of inclusion is pivotal. To my mind, the discussions about human rights and occupational justice taking place amongst occupational therapists (WFOT 2019) chart a path that leads straight to inclusion, and to recognition that promoting inclusion is the single most important thing that the profession can contribute to society. Perhaps it is all we contribute, for what use is enhanced function if it does not lead to children playing and learning with their peers, and people with disabilities, including cognitive decline, living on equal terms with others? Why work in hospitals, community centres, residential care settings, housing services, workplaces, prisons; with people living in poverty, refugee camps or disaster zones; with sports groups, local councils, employers, architects, benefactors and politicians – if not to shift the balance towards visibility, acceptance and inclusion of all members of society?

Inclusion is now the cornerstone of occupational therapy curricula. To promote that vision, the World Federation of Occupational Therapists (WFOT) (2016, p.5) calls us 'to engage in community capacity building and societal change.' Educators are directed to 'advance social participation, health, wellness and social inclusion globally with knowledge and practices that address the social determinants of health and occupational justice, beyond education on bodily dysfunction', with an end goal of 'building a more peaceful, prosperous and just world' (WFOT 2016, p.11). This will be achieved by upholding 'principles of dignity, equality and equity', contributing to research on occupation, as well as social participation and inclusion, human rights and 'the "enablement" of populations, communities and individuals' (p.11). All these elements are represented in this book. Chapters span individual perspectives on life with dementia and fostering personal relationships, through to brain health, social transformation and issues of occupational justice. Equally, the occupationally focused interventions described extend from self-management, engaging with digital technologies and memory rehabilitation to rights-based practice and participation in research. Throughout, there is a sense of people with dementia coming first amongst professionals and family carers, with an emphasis given to active engagement and being accorded the right, dignity and responsibility of co-designing interventions and generating knowledge.

Occupational therapists are not alone in championing people with dementia as citizens and active participants in their own lives. In August 2021, the World Health Organization (WHO) launched its toolkit to promote the social inclusion of people with dementia by raising awareness and understanding of dementia and scaling up dementia-friendly initiatives (WHO 2021b). Like occupational therapists, their goal is to ensure that people with dementia can remain in and be part of their communities. As I've argued, occupational therapists have an active role to play in this. Promoting inclusion means we must look beyond exclusionary processes, including ageism, discrimination, stigmatization and the barriers experienced by people with dementia. We don't need more information about the problems encountered. It is already well recognized that people with dementia can be excluded from decisions made by family members (however well meaning), about finances, continuing to drive, accessing healthcare, participating in social activities and living independently. We know that people with dementia can become socially isolated, as others shy away from declining abilities rather than supporting continued engagement. We also already know that risk aversion and a focus on physical harm restricts the occupations accessible to residents in care facilities (British Society of Gerontology 2020). Rather than this negative stance, occupational therapists are well placed to forge alliances with people with dementia, to learn from them what inclusion means from their perspective, what it feels like, how they want to be included and how inclusion can be promoted.

Research employing an occupational perspective is generating new knowledge that will inform us, and others, about ways to communicate and 'be with' people with dementia. For example, when diminished language skills make communication complex, Tatzer's (2019) work with narratives-in-action can help us learn to 'read' the meanings people with dementia convey through the things they do. Even when the narrative has become fragmented, efforts to recognize consistent elements in people's actions and self-presentation can reveal much about their identity and social roles. Thus, one of Tatzer's participants conveyed much about her recent life, interests and responsibilities when she retrieved a collection of ornamental angels from her voluminous handbag, and proceeded to position, clean and display them. These were beloved reminders of life before entering residential care and her responsibilities as a custodian of a community garden inhabited by more than 140 garden angels. Similarly, Kielsgaard and colleagues used a narrative-in-action approach to initiate and accompany residents in a dementia town as they walked around, interacting with the people encountered and the environment (Kielsgaard *et al.* 2021). The researchers came to appreciate one resident as a postman who took great pride in walking the city and skilfully holding the letters for delivery and another as returning to a favoured role, shopping with her girlfriends. These moments of shared meaning, enjoyment and appreciation of each other, experienced through shared occupation, are precious and accessible. Like the 'switch-on' effect observed amongst participants in cognitive stimulation programmes (Liu, Jones and Hocking 2020), they seem to be accessed through doing pleasant things together in non-threatening contexts.

Supporting that vision, the editors of *Occupational Therapy and Dementia: Promoting Inclusion, Rights and Opportunities for People Living with Dementia* have assembled the best of occupational therapy practice at this time, with each chapter contributing to an overall picture of the possibilities opening up for people with dementia and their caregivers. This is a far cry from the 'accepted' truths of last century's dementia care. Applying an occupational perspective to practice has broad-ranging impact, not least by placing emphasis on enhancing the lives of people with dementia through engagement in occupation and showing participation to be an achievable goal. Bringing occupation into the conversation confirms the centrality of person-centred care and co-design of services, because each person's occupational priorities and meanings are unique, and services must be responsive to that if they are to be effective. An occupational perspective also brings to light the fact that the occupational possibilities available to people exist within societal structures that determine access to therapy, the provision of assistive technologies, daily routines, resources, staffing levels, attitudes and priorities in residential care facilities. Occupational therapists must be alert to those influences and armed with knowledge to break down attitudinal and environmental barriers. Most important, when we view the world through an occupational lens, issues of occupational justice and inclusion surface and must be addressed. The topics covered in this book – rights-based education and practice – declare that as a profession we are more than equipped to pick up the challenge.

References

British Society of Gerontology (2020) 'Social inclusion of people with dementia.' Blog, 14 February. Accessed on 10/10/2021 at https://ageingissues.wordpress.com/2020/02/14/social-inclusion-of-people-with-dementia

Friedell, M. (2003) 'Remarks to Ventura.' Paper presentation, Annual Education Conference of the California Central Coast Alzheimer's Association, California.

Kielsgaard, K., Horghagen, S., Nielsen, D. and Kristensen, H.K. (2021) 'Moments of meaning: Enacted narratives of occupational engagement within a dementia town.' *Journal of Occupational Science 28*, 4, 510–524. Accessed on 22/04/2022 at https://doi.org/10.1080/14427591.2020.1859403

Liu, Q., Jones, M. and Hocking, C. (2020) 'Describing and measuring the "switch-on" effect in people with dementia who participate in cognitive stimulation therapy: A mixed methods study.' *British Journal of Occupational Therapy 83*, 5, 316–325. Accessed on 22/04/2022 at https://doi.org/10.1177/0308022619899301

O'Sullivan, G. and Hocking, C. (2013) 'Translating action research into practice: Seeking occupational justice for people with dementia.' *OTJR: Occupation, Participation and Health 33*, 3, 168–176. Accessed on 22/04/2022 at https://doi.org/10.3928/15394492-20130614-05

O'Sullivan, G., Hocking, C. and Spence, D. (2014a) 'Action research: Changing history for people with dementia in New Zealand.' *Action Research 12*, 1, 19–35. Accessed on 22/04/2022 at https://doi.org/10.1177/1476750313509417

O'Sullivan, G., Hocking, C. and Spence, D. (2014b) 'Dementia: The need for attitudinal change'. *Dementia: The International Journal of Social Research and Practice 13*, 4, 483–497. Accessed on 22/04/2022 at https://doi.org/10.1177/1471301213478241

Tatzer, V.C. (2019) 'Narratives-in-action of people with moderate to severe dementia in long-term care: Understanding the link between occupation and identity.' *Journal of Occupational Science 26*, 2, 245–257. Accessed on 22/04/2022 at https://doi.org/1 0.1080/14427591.2019.1600159

Taylor, R. (2007) *Alzheimer's from the Inside Out*. Baltimore, MD: Health Profession Press.

WFOT (World Federation of Occupational Therapists) (2016) *Minimum Standards for the Education of Occupational Therapists 2016*. London: WFOT. Accessed on 10/10/2021 at www.wfot.org/resources/new-minimum-standards-for-the-education-of-occupational-therapists-2016-e-copy

WFOT (2019) *Occupational Therapy and Human Rights (Revised)*. Position Statement. London: WFOT. Accessed on 10/10/2021 at www.wfot.org/resources/occupational-therapy-and-human-rights

WHO (World Health Organization) (2021a) 'Dementia.' Fact sheets, 2 September. Geneva: WHO. Accessed on 25/11/2021 at www.who.int/news-room/fact-sheets/detail/dementia

WHO (2021b) 'New WHO toolkit promotes inclusion of people with dementia in society.' News, 6 August. Geneva: WHO. Accessed on 10/10/2021 at www.who.int/news/item/06-08-2021-who-launches-new-toolkit-to-promote-dementia-inclusive-societies

Professor Clare Hocking, Department of Occupational Science and Therapy, Auckland University of Technology, Tāmaki Makaurau Auckland, Aotearoa New Zealand

CHAPTER I

Introduction

Fiona Maclean, Alison Warren, Elaine Hunter and Lyn Westcott

When you looked at this book for the first time, you may have noticed the embroidery of the brain. This is by one of our authors (Lorna) who had a CT scan to confirm her diagnosis of dementia and did not understand what the image was telling her. She used her long-standing interest in creative embroidery to help her come to terms with her diagnosis, and to understand the personal meaning of this. The starting inspiration for our introduction to you is the combination of Lorna's CT scan, her embroidery skills and how she valued this occupation.

We, the editors of this book, have connected at different times in our occupational therapy careers. For example, Fiona and Elaine worked together in an older adult service in Scotland; Alison and Fiona presented at the same Occupational Science conference; Lyn and Alison worked together as occupational therapy educators; and Elaine and Lyn sat together on the Royal College of Occupational Therapists (RCOT) Board for Learning and Development at the same time. It was Fiona who brought us together through our shared passion for occupational therapy, dementia and the difference we know the profession can make to people's lives every day.

We wanted to inspire our occupational therapists of today, tomorrow and the future to be leaders, innovators, researchers and rights-based practitioners in dementia. We also all bring a very personal perspective of dementia that has inspired our thinking, creation and writing of this book. In editing this book for you, we knew we wanted to have the person with dementia and their caregivers to guide and inspire you, and it was important to have the voice of lived experience at the start of the book (see Chapters 2 and 3). We have chosen the term 'caregiver' throughout the text to refer to family members and informal carers supporting people living with dementia. To maintain confidentiality, we use pseudonyms in case examples to represent aspects of work known to the authors, although specific details are excluded.

The contributors to this book bring a wide range of perspectives that explore the right to and the importance of meaningful occupation in daily life for all. There are also contributions from a variety of professionals working alongside occupational therapists who make an equally important difference to people's lives. Occupational therapists from practice, academia and research share their insights and practical approaches. This mix is essential to illustrate how best evidence and current knowledge can be mobilized and translated into occupational therapy dementia practice. With over 40 contributors, we, as editors, recognize the value of the original writing styles of authorship teams, to encourage people to reveal their experience. We see this as a strength of the text.

We wanted a book that shared the ground-breaking work of many of our occupational therapists, partners and friends to inspire, challenge and encourage you at all times to be a rights-based practitioner. Whilst we have shared an occupational perspective from UK national and international authors, we also acknowledge that not all current work in occupational therapy and dementia is included simply because we did not have the scope to cover it all. Our passion in editing this book for you recognizes that whatever your chosen area of occupational therapy, you will meet people living with dementia and their caregivers. Consequently, we invite you in your practice to be curious, bold and inspired, and importantly to truly listen to the person's narrative with grace and ease. Be committed to then walk alongside the person as and when they share their occupational journey with you.

The need for this book

As you work with people living with dementia, your professional commitment will increasingly be influenced by the necessity to recognize how, and in what way, a human rights-based approach can influence your practice. The Universal Declaration of Human Rights (UN General Assembly 1948) is widely regarded as a core foundation of understanding. This outlines that all humans, regardless of who we are or where we come from, are afforded the right to dignity, equality, fairness and respect, to have their freedom protected and their autonomy engendered, which will allow people to direct their own lives.

A global perspective of human rights informing policy directing health and social care is increasingly visible. In addition, the debate around the equitable access to participation in occupations identified as important by people and groups, as a human right (Whalley Hammell 2008), has been positioned as a central focus of concern for the profession. Yet often the translation of a human rights-based approach from theory and/or policy to everyday practice can remain unclear – in part because complex cultural, political and organizational systems exist alongside growing inequalities of health. As such, it can be difficult to influence a professional response alongside these high-level factors, which can be seen as restrictive to change. Moreover, subtle and nuanced variations in the interpretation of human rights can coexist from person to person, practice context to practice context, nation to nation. Nevertheless, the need for occupational therapists to feel empowered to advocate for the rights of people living with dementia has never been more needed, because these rights can often be overlooked. People living with dementia frequently experience stigma and unequal opportunity to rehabilitation, or are excluded from decision-making that often impacts life-changing transitions.

To uphold, affirm and promote respect for the rights of people living with dementia, their families and caregivers, the World Health Organization (WHO) (2015) notes the importance of the PANEL framework. The acronym of PANEL forefronts five concepts that can aid the translation of a rights-based approach to practice. These are:

- *Participation:* Everyone has the right to participate in decisions that affect them.
- *Accountability:* There should be effective monitoring of human rights standards, as well as effective mechanisms of response when breached.
- *Non-discrimination:* Discrimination in all forms in the realization of rights must be prohibited, prevented and eliminated.
- *Empowerment:* People and communities should understand their rights and be fully supported to participate in the development of policy and practices that affect their lives.
- *Legality:* Rights as legally enforceable entitlements, linked

> to national and international human rights law, should be recognized. (Alzheimer Scotland 2021)

As occupational therapists are increasingly called on to advocate for and remain vigilant of the need to protect the everyday rights of people living with dementia, PANEL offers a mechanism of response. By embedding the principles of PANEL into professional practice, occupational therapists increase the likelihood of ensuring people living with dementia sustain their right to remain socially connected, as part of communities, and able to maintain their identity and sense of purpose through valued activity. A starting premise of this book, therefore, is that all people living with dementia have the right to a personal life, including the right to live independently and to be included in any decisions made about and with them.

The requirement to respect the human rights of people living with dementia is universal. The various chapters throughout this book therefore offer examples of the opportunities in which therapists can act in practice to galvanize the rights of people living with dementia. In addition, each chapter offers scope for critical reflection, to identify, question and explore assumptions that may exist, including knowledge of dementia. Thus, one goal of this book is to re-energize how occupational therapy students and graduates think about dementia, thereby influencing how we act in practice.

Structure of the book

Nevertheless, the juxtaposition of a human rights-based approach and an occupation-focused theoretical lens that 'drives' everyday practice can be perplexing. On the one hand, there is clear and evolving discussion promoting the need to be cognisant of occupational justice and injustice emerging from occupational science. This contrasts with the tendency of practitioners towards the adoption of conceptual models that can act to guide and direct everyday practice. The intersection between the study of humans as occupational beings, set within the social and political contexts in which practice occurs, guided by the essential need to retain occupation as core to professional contribution, was a point of consideration in the development of this text.

We opted for pragmatism. Whilst the chapters in and of themselves offer examples of how and in what way the profession can respond to and reflect on a human rights-based approach to dementia practice, the structure of the text is framed by the themes of 'person', 'environment' and 'occupation'. The seminal work of Law *et al.* (1996) has been influential in our thinking because working with people living with dementia, their families and caregivers can be complex. It requires us to understand that our involvement with the person, their environment and their occupations will never remain static. It is instead a dynamic, transactional relationship that is further influenced by the constant ebb and flow of shifting theory and science, influencing practice.

In adopting the themes of 'person', 'environment' and 'occupation', Figure 1.1 illustrates their overarching interdependence by assuming a semi-permeable membrane that can 'breathe' in and out, between and within these themes, to encompass the wider context, influences and experiences of people living with dementia, their families and caregivers, steering towards an occupation-focused, rights-based approach to practice. As such, the chapters have been positioned under person, environment and occupation through editorial discussion of where we felt author contributions may best correspond. This is not to say that some chapters could not be placed elsewhere, bridging across and between person–environment–occupation.

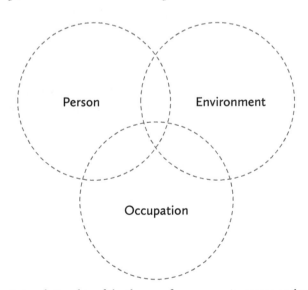

Figure 1.1. Interrelationship of the themes of person, environment and occupation

How to use this book

Set within this context, we hope that you will enjoy this book and want to read it from cover to cover. That said, we know that people engage in books in different ways. Books should meet the needs of the reader, and these will vary depending on your knowledge and understanding, interest in the content and contributors, and perhaps your work or study role and what you wish to learn alongside your current level of expertise. The book, as noted above, is divided into three sections with chapters that share a common focus. Chapters 2–5 are grouped under the theme of 'person', Chapters 6–10 'environment' and 11–17 'occupation'.

It may be that as you look at a chapter in the book, others in that section will feel relevant for you. We have tried to make some in-text links between the chapters, to help you navigate around relevant contributions and themes. The index will also help you find a discussion of topics included in several chapters. Whatever way you decide to select your reading, please ensure that you look at the learning outcomes that all contributors have put at the start of their chapters. These help to indicate what the content is about, and what you may achieve by engaging with the material. Subheadings will help you to scan through the chapter, so you can find discussion linked to specific learning outcomes more easily, if you do not wish to read the whole chapter, although we would, of course, recommend that you do! The contributors have spent time outlining some helpful reflective questions at the end of each chapter. These are to help you apply and engage the concepts you have just read about, alongside reflecting on your own experiences and ideas on how occupational therapists may work with people living with dementia and their caregivers. We would advise keeping those reflections to revisit another day. This will help you evaluate your own professional development, and as your reasoning becomes more influenced by a rights-based approach, it will lead to deeper learning and enhanced professional occupational therapy practice.

We hope that this book will be helpful in supporting your study in dementia, occupational therapy and rights-based working.

References

Alzheimer Scotland (2021) 'Rights based approach to dementia.' Edinburgh: Alzheimer Scotland. Accessed on 20/12/2021 at www.alzscot.org/our-work/campaigning-for-change/rights-based-approach-to-dementia

Law, M., Cooper, B.A., Strong, S., Stewart, D., Rigby, P. and Letts, L. (1996) 'The person–environment–occupation model: A transactive approach to occupational performance.' *Canadian Journal of Occupational Therapy 63*, 1, 9–23.

UN (United Nations) General Assembly (1948) *Universal Declaration of Human Rights* (217 A [III]). Paris: UN. Accessed on 24/11/2021 at www.un.org/en/about-us/universal-declaration-of-human-rights

Whalley Hammell, K. (2008) 'Reflections on...well-being and occupational rights.' *Canadian Journal of Occupational Therapy 75*, 1, 61–64.

WHO (World Health Organization) (2015) *Ensuring a Human Rights-Based Approach for People Living with Dementia.* Geneva: WHO. Accessed on 20/12/2021 at www.ohchr.org/sites/default/files/Documents/Issues/OlderPersons/Dementia/ThematicBrief.pdf

PERSON

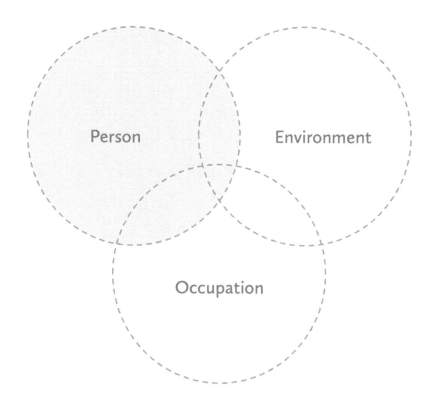

CHAPTER 2

The Voices of People Living with Dementia

Anthony Schrag, Henry Rankin, Lorna Noble,
Margaret McCallion and Wendy Rankin

Learning outcomes

By the end of this chapter, you will have the opportunity to:

▶ Reflect on the value and power of including and listening to the voice(s) of people living with dementia to influence the priorities and focus of occupational therapy service delivery
▶ Recognize the significance of the contribution self-advocacy groups such as the Scottish Dementia Working Group (SDWG) can offer to campaign for and on behalf of people living with dementia
▶ Explore how and in what ways creativity remains central to the lives of three particular members of the SDWG, and how this positively influences their ability to live well with dementia
▶ Consider how these three, shared stories can influence and reshape your existing practice.

Introduction

As early as 1997 Tom Kitwood presented the need for a paradigm of understanding in which the person living with dementia should come first. Since this early work, people with lived experience of dementia increasingly inform professional understanding of the impact of this diagnosis on their everyday lives, such as Agnes Houston and Julie Christie (2018), Wendy Mitchell (2018) and Kate Swaffer (2021). Their personal experiences, shared via social media, conference presentations and contributions to professional education, offer an invaluable insight for those who work with people living with dementia, including occupational therapists. As such, this opening chapter begins by introducing and explaining the role and purpose of the Scottish Dementia Working Group (SDWG), of which all members must have a diagnosis of dementia. Three members of the SDWG, Margaret, Henry and Lorna, go on to share their unique experiences of living with dementia as described to Anthony, one of the co-authors of this chapter. Their separate conversations with Anthony are summarized and presented here to give insight into the value and importance of creativity and occupation when living with dementia.

Scottish Dementia Working Group

The SDWG is a national, member-led campaigning and awareness-raising group for people living with a diagnosis of dementia in Scotland. Funded by Alzheimer Scotland and the Scottish Government, the SDWG is the independent voice of people living with dementia in Scotland. Over recent years, the SDWG has significantly influenced professional education, working in partnership with occupational therapy interns and supporting innovative practice education (see also Chapter 10).

The SDWG prides itself on being a friendly and inclusive group led by, and for, people with dementia, and has a dedicated staff team who help facilitate and support the group's activities. Anyone living in Scotland with a diagnosis of dementia is welcome to join, and the only requirement for membership is that members are happy to meet other people with dementia to discuss things that matter to them. For families, there are similar groups including the National Dementia Carers Action Network (NDCAN) in Scotland and Together in Dementia Everyday (TIDE) in England and Scotland.

Although the SDWG is not a formal support group, member feedback has indicated that those who join have gained support and have made friends through their membership. Since the SDWG was established in 2001, it has gone from strength to strength, and has represented a collective voice for people with lived experience of dementia, campaigning and raising awareness at both a national and local level. SDWG members have travelled far and wide to tell their stories, speaking at conferences and events across the world to help raise awareness of dementia and to challenge stigma. Many members have written impactful blogs sharing their experiences of issues such as receiving a diagnosis, having younger onset dementia and becoming a campaigner.

The SDWG regularly works with a range of stakeholders nationally and across communities to engage with and inform recent Scottish Government National Dementia Strategies. They have presented and shared their experiences of having dementia with many health and social care professionals. Over the years they have been involved in areas such as housing, technology, transport and research. As one member said so eloquently, 'We all do something; we don't just sit on our hands and let the world pass us by.'

This commitment to influence, change and challenge public and professional perceptions of what it is to live with dementia led three members of the SDWG, Margaret, Henry and Lorna, to share their experiences of living with dementia for this book. The nature and meaning of creativity as part of their lives was chosen as the focus of their conversation with Anthony. This was mutually agreed due to the value placed on creativity as a foundation of occupational therapy practice, including its wider potential to bring people together.

Creativity and other people

Philosopher Emmanuel Levinas (1989) suggested that as social creatures, human beings can only ever truly learn about themselves by engaging with others. Encountering someone different from oneself, however, can sometimes be difficult because it means we have to reconcile our own individualized existence within a wider social context. Being exposed to an 'other' and understanding them as a fully-formed, complex, nuanced being with histories, ideas and politics is a hard thing to do, and it is therefore sometimes easier to distil these people into more simplistic categories. We think: this person is my lecturer; that person is a politician; here is someone living with dementia. These categories are useful to help us get through the day, but they do not provide any chance for deeper understanding of others, or of ourselves. For example, the lecturer might also be a mother of three children, who loves nothing more than playing poker online; the politician might love Mexican food and be fond of growing plants; and the person living with dementia might be a critically acclaimed filmmaker, as well as having a secret love of glam rock. Knowing these nuances of an individual allows us to further relate to these people – we can speak to the lecturer about poker strategies; we can share tips for seeding begonias; we can toe-tap along to T. Rex's track 'Hot Love'. Knowing the creative passions of someone else helps us learn and adapt to them in the same way they might learn and adapt to our own particular individual peculiarities.

Conceptually, this is not difficult to understand – we all *know* other people have rich inner lives and histories with complex emotions and thoughts, but keeping this at the forefront of our mind and *living* this knowledge without reducing people to a two-dimensional version of themselves is a much harder activity, particularly when working along-side those living with a disease that complicates their own identities.

Whilst this book does not aim to suggest anyone can possibly understand the entirety of someone's complex inner life, it does hope to indicate that there might be some key themes that can begin to give rich insights in to who someone is. For example, talking about family and work can reveal central truths about who the person is, what they love and what is important to them. These are not, however, universal themes and they are not without hidden dangers – veering into the choppy waters of complex family relationships might, for some, be more traumatic than productive.

Another central theme that perhaps avoids such pitfalls is creativity. Creativity is, after all, essential to the human condition. Anthropologist Agustín Fuentes (2017) argues that creativity is one of the main traits that make us successful both as a species, and also as individuals. Importantly, creativity does not mean art. It does not mean painting, drawing or acting. Certainly for some, these might be vital elements of their identity, but creativity generally relates to the ways in which people express themselves: a footballer can be creative in how she kicks that ball, which shows her love for the game and her unique talents; a bicycle courier can be creative in the route he takes to deliver the next package to go down his favourite hill; the sister experiments with a vegan cake to show her love for her ecologically minded brother. These are all examples of the ability of humans to be creative and find ways to express the things that are important to them. Creativity, then, like occupation, is a mechanism of expression of values, and is best defined as a 'Central source of meaning in our lives...most of the things that are interesting, important, and human are the results of creativity... [and] when we are involved in it, we feel that we are living more fully than during the rest of life' (Csikszentmihalyi 2013, p.1). By extension, professional curiosity of the relationship between the concept of flow and occupation (Emerson 1998) can also be helpful to our understanding of the wider value of creativity.

Below, we explore the creativity central to three members of the SDWG: Margaret, a retired directorate administrator, Henry, a retired police officer, and Lorna, a retired primary school headteacher. As short snippets of their lives, these narratives provide a brief insight into the different ways to explore how central creativity has been in their own self-identity, self-worth and meaning-making. We hope they can provide an insight into the centrality of creative expression in understanding someone else, to influence the ways we shape our practice.

MARGARET

Margaret logs on to the online meeting a bit flustered; a previous meeting had run late, and her computer was acting up. She politely apologizes, settles into her chair, smooths down her dress and instantly wins everyone over with a bright smile and a wee joke. She exudes a sense of calm and efficiency, ready to take on the world.

This snippet of life – the complications of online life – is a common-enough experience for all of us in the 'COVID-times' when this occurred, and seems to capture the core part of Margaret: that despite difficulties (a global pandemic), she has continued to be quintessentially 'herself' – adaptable, bright and with a no-nonsense approach that has an edge of fun. It is an approach that serves her well as part of the SDWG and the European Working Group of People with Dementia with whom she volunteers. It is important to her to feel useful, and to contribute to these demanding groups is a central part of who she is; despite the restrictions of the past year, she has managed to adapt these commitments to the online world.

Indeed, this work and the global restrictions imposed on us all haven't stopped Margaret from enjoying her creative passion: music. She tells us that she has always sung, and before she was diagnosed, she was into amateur dramatics, was cantor at church, and has even been in a rock choir. Pre-COVID-19 there was a singing group that took place next to the SDWG cafe, where musicians Cappella Nova led weekly music workshops with people with dementia. As well as this group, she is also in the Scottish Opera Community Choir, where they sing in four-part harmonies, which she 'thoroughly enjoys'. Even during lockdown it was important for her to participate in these creative activities. She has taken weekly sessions online, and whilst this is not ideal, it has been central to her wellbeing:

> It's enjoyable when we're singing a song. What's not so enjoyable are the warm-ups before, and whilst I've always enjoyed warm-ups, when you're doing it yourself, singing it yourself in your room, your family thinks you're going insane, [especially] when we're doing siren sounds and things.

We all have a giggle at the thought of her warbling siren sounds, alone in her room, whilst her family outside look perplexed at the strange sounds emanating from behind a closed door.

It's not just about singing, though: music is a central part of who she is. She says:

> I've always loved music. I was used to going out to theatres or going to concerts, you know, but I just always have enjoyed music. At home – obviously not when I'm on a meeting! – I've always got the radio on. I love my radio.

She likes all sorts of music, too: 'I love Motown; I love a lot the music from the 80s; I love musicals. I also like some soft rock stuff as well...' She pauses and reflects, and with a wry smile, says: 'I don't like country music... Okay, I have liked some of the country songs I've heard, but couldn't listen to a whole country music programme.' Her laughter is light and songlike.

When asked about the centrality of music in her life, she's quite clear: it provides meaning to her life in the same way as her family, friends and work. When asked what it would mean to not be able to enjoy it – what it would mean if someone did not understand how important it is to her – she goes quiet, and it's the first time she doesn't have the smile lines on her face. Her voice is serious and clear, and she adjusts herself in her seat and says: 'Um...I think there used to be a song called "When the Music Died"...that, I think that that would upset me.' She doesn't shy away from difficult or uncomfortable subjects, but prefers to focus on what can be done practically, and so she helpfully offers a solution: 'I think the most important thing is always make sure you see the person as a person... Maybe that's not that easy to do, but people with dementia don't all have the same symptoms or illnesses.' Nor, she recognizes, do they have the same passions and interests. For Margaret, she's not just a person with dementia; she's also a creative individual whose particular creativity manifests in her love of music.

HENRY

Henry smiles through the computer screen and says: 'I'm just Henry. I am still the same person. I can't change it.' This openness to speak about his diagnosis is a hallmark of his honesty and frankness, and is part of the reason he has worked with the SDWG for 13 years and has even been its chairperson. He's also on the Board of Trustees with Alzheimer Scotland and is a Dementia Champion at the University of the West of Scotland, helping in the education of student nurses and allied health professionals.

He's therefore well known in the field, and people speak fondly of him because they've known him for so long. When we speak to him, however, he wryly lets us in on a secret: he loves cowboy films. A colleague is surprised; they've known him for many, many years, but did not know this about him. Henry gives a cheeky grin, content to have surprised someone. Again.

Henry explains that his love of cowboy films first started when he was very young. His mother sent him to the cinema, saying 'You'll like this'...and she was right, he did! He's spent most of his life enjoying these films, and it doesn't matter if he's seen a film a thousand times, he will still watch it. When asked why, he explains that it's because they always get their man: no matter the risks, and no matter how terrible the adversary, or how many people he was up against, the cowboy always won, and they 'never get beat with anything'. They always had a plan, and they always got the bad guy and saved the girl.

The quintessential cowboy was John Wayne in the white hat. Cowboys had a moral compass and the strength to *do the right thing*. It's no surprise, then, that Henry was a police officer for many decades, and he says, with a twinkle in his eye, that he sees a direct correlation between his passion for cowboys and his chosen career. He jokes, however, that he sees one distinct difference: 'police officers didn't have guns'. But he says he did enjoy the work, because it was about 'the good guys getting the bad guys'.

When he started policing, Henry says that getting into the police force was difficult, with exams and training...but he surprised himself by passing all of the exams with flying colours. He then worked in the force for decades, including places like the Gorbals (an area in the city of Glasgow, Scotland) in the 1960s and 1970s – which were known to be difficult places to work. But he loved it, if only because it was very social: he got to speak to people, and it was important to have those relationships with the regular 'characters'. He enjoyed having a 'blether and just a chitchat', which helped him understand his community and the area. He reflects and says it was the 'right job' for him, and he has no regrets about it. And it wasn't just policing and cowboys; he also played football, playing for the 'F' division, enjoying the rivalry with the local 'G' division – and he proudly speaks of their annual match that they only lost once, something that decades later still makes him smile.

It's clear that Henry is not shy when talking about his past and the things that give his life meaning. He talks openly about his diagnosis, in much the same way he used to love talking to people on his police beat. He's open, friendly and engaging. He says the worst thing to happen with someone living with dementia is to 'be put in a corner', to be defined through their diagnosis alone, and this is why he volunteers with the SDWG and is a Dementia Champion. He knows that not everyone can advocate for those living with dementia, and he's not going to let his diagnosis stop him from 'fighting the good fight'.

Letting us in on the secret of his love for cowboy films gives us a deeper insight into the quintessential nature of 'Henry'. Whilst it could be seen as just a pastime or a passing interest, his engagement with this creative medium – cowboy films – can also be a further way to understand Henry as a whole person, what drives him, what he is passionate about, and what gives his life meaning and purpose.

LORNA

Lorna says she'd like to embroider her brain. This sounds confusing at first: what does she mean? How would one do that? Is it even safe?! Stepping back and looking at this in context, it all starts to make sense.

Lorna is an impressive woman. She was a primary school head-teacher for a number of years, and so knows her way around people – she is gentle, but firm, and like all good educators, she is encouraging and wise. It is uplifting to talk to her, and when speaking to her online, you can see bright, colourful pictures crowding together on the wall behind her whilst the sunshine streams through the window.

The images around her are her own artworks. She's always been interested in looking at art, but as 'a headteacher, there was not time for your own things', so she never had much time to explore her own creativity. When she retired, however, a chance opportunity opened a whole new world for her. At the time she was living in Cornwall and a local college offered an access course to art and design classes – £10 for an entire year to take a variety of different classes and activities – and she thought, 'why not?'

She admits that when she started the classes, she had little experience in art-making: 'As a primary school teacher, you're a jack of all trades and a master of none, you teach everything.' But the classes offered her a chance to learn about printing, felting, pottery, painting and art history, to name just a few. She discovered that not only was she quite good, but she actually got an immense amount of pleasure from these works. She found not only a way to creatively express herself, but also a community. She joined a felting group and an embroidery group, and over the years took part in various exhibitions.

You can see the pride and joy in her eyes when she talks about her works, and her artwork is a way to understand her more. She holds up an example to the camera, and a blur of muted colours flows over the screen, slowly revealing itself to be an Orcadian Island scene: North Ronaldsay. There is a sturdy, shining lighthouse on a craggy shore off to the right; the grey-blues of the North Atlantic rush the middle of the canvas, as if you could hear the waves; and the famous North Ronaldsay sheep munch on the greenie-brown seaweed that gives their meat that wonderful flavour. The work is electric, and looking at it for longer you realize that it is a collage comprising different materials, some painted, some felt and some embroidered, and to complete the frieze, an embroidered map of the island.

Lorna says she wants to give it away to the bird sanctuary on the island: 'I don't have any family here, by choice and age. And I have Alzheimer's, so I don't know how long I'm going to live, so I want it to go somewhere good and somewhere that will appreciate it.' She explains that the island is where her grandfather is from, and so donating to this place is a connection she can make with her past; like the threads she joins together when felting, the past, present and future are also joined together in this beautiful work.

It's a beautiful gesture that's mirrored in her statement that she wants to embroider her brain. She means, of course, that she would like to embroider an image of the scan of her brain. She says that the image was so unique and interesting that she would like to explore that through her craft.

It is a brave act to focus her attention on the thing that confirmed her diagnosis and the uniqueness of her condition. It is obvious, however, that Lorna would find it empowering too: it is a way of exploring the meaning of her context, to understand and express herself in relation to her condition. In this way, making this new artwork is not *only* a creative act of self-expression, it also provides meaning through occupation, context and insight, both for Lorna herself, and for those who then see her works.

Spending any time with Lorna will reveal what an interesting person she is; however, the artworks she makes are a shorthand that can provide a much deeper insight into who she is. Like her artworks, she is bright, brave, generous, unique and colourful. What would it mean to her if she could not participate in such creative acts?

Conclusion

In this chapter, we have considered the value and power of including and listening to the voice(s) of people living with dementia every day to influence your priorities and focus as an occupational therapist. We have shared three stories that we hope will influence and reshape your existing practice, and help you to recognize that by being creative, you can positively influence a person's life to live well with dementia.

We invited our three 'storytellers' to answer this question:

What is the most important thing occupational therapists need to think about when it comes to people with dementia?

They replied:

I think when you're doing something with dementia, if you didn't know what it is...you should try and find out. (Henry)

I think the important thing is that I'm still me, even though I have Alzheimer's. (Lorna)

No matter what the diagnosis is, always make sure you see the person as a person. (Margaret)

Reflective questions

1. Having read these short narratives, what practical steps might you take to enhance and explore the creativity of someone living with dementia?
2. In what ways can you explore the creativity of someone living with dementia, including as a way to build relationships?
3. Have a look on different digital platforms and read through the blogs, tweets and podcasts where people living with dementia are sharing their stories with honesty and passion. What are your experiences of this?

Acknowledgements

We would like to acknowledge the valuable contribution of two occupational therapy students who were on placement with the SDWG, and who helped us to share these narratives: Claire Wilkie and Gill O'Shaughnessy.

References

Csikszentmihalyi, M. (2013) *Creativity: The Psychology of Discovery and Invention.* New York: Harper Perennial Modern Classics.

Emerson, H. (1998) 'Flow and occupation: A review of the literature.' *Canadian Journal of Occupational Therapy 65*, 1, 37–43.

Fuentes, A. (2017) *The Creative Spark: How Imagination Made Humans Exceptional.* London: Dutton Books.

Houston, A. and Christie, J. (2018) *Talking Sense: Living with Sensory Changes in Dementia.* Sydney, NSW: Australia Hammond Care.

Kitwood, T. (1997) *Dementia Reconsidered: The Person Comes First.* Buckingham: Open University Press.

Levinas, E. (ed.) (1989) *The Levinas Reader* (edited by S. Hand). Oxford: Blackwell.

Mitchell, W. (2018) *Somebody I Used to Know.* London: Bloomsbury.

Swaffer, K. (2021) 'Rehabilitation: A Human Right for Everyone.' In L.F. Low and K. Laver (eds) *Dementia Rehabilitation: Evidence-Based Interventions and Clinical Recommendations* (Chapter 1). London: Elsevier.

CHAPTER 3

Always Looking for a Solution

Chris Roberts and Jayne Goodrick in
Conversation with Alison Warren

Chris Roberts, Jayne Goodrick and Alison Warren

> ### Learning outcomes
> By the end of this chapter, you will have the opportunity to:
>
> ▶ Gain insights into how taking practical problem-solving approaches, keeping active, busy and learning new skills can be part of a person's life when living with dementia
> ▶ Recognize the importance of upholding the rights of people living with dementia and their families
> ▶ Consider through reflection how the information shared from conversations between Chris, Jayne and Alison may influence your practice.

About the authors

Chris Roberts lives in North Wales with his wife, Jayne Goodrick, and their children. He is a motorbike enthusiast with a passion for customizing bespoke high-performance motorbikes, and he enjoyed attending rallies. Chris has balanced a variety of roles including father, motorbike shop owner and working in sales and property maintenance. Chris was diagnosed with vascular dementia and later Alzheimer's disease in his early fifties, and is approaching his sixtieth birthday.

Jayne Goodrick has known Chris since high school, and they married in 1994. They share a common interest in motorbikes, travel and adventures in their motorhome. Jayne has studied Chinese metaphysics. She first noticed a change in Chris approximately ten years ago.

Some of you may be aware of elements of Chris and Jayne's story from a BBC Panorama television programme that was aired in the UK in 2016.

Alison Warren is an occupational therapist with a keen interest in supporting people living with dementia of all ages and their caregivers. Early in her career she was alarmed by the lack of consideration of the occupational needs of people, and became involved in occupation-focused service developments and research. Alison met Jayne and Chris several years ago and was aware that sharing insights from their practical experience of living with dementia would be a great learning opportunity for occupational therapists and students.

Introduction

This is Chris and Jayne's story.

I (Alison) had the privilege of spending some time in conversation with Chris and Jayne to try to capture insights into their life pre-'dementiaville' (Jayne's term) and the routes their journey has taken them on since diagnosis. From the outset, Chris and Jayne were clear that they wanted to be involved with this book, although they preferred me to collate their experiences, hence the co-authorship approach taken with this chapter.

I first met Chris and Jayne at a Prime Minister's Dementia Challenge Group for Air Transport based at the Civil Aviation Authority (CAA) headquarters in London in 2018. As the chairperson went around the room facilitating introductions, as always, I introduced myself as an occupational therapist, now working at a university with occupational therapy students and undertaking research. I heard a sound to my side and Chris caught my eye. Not sure what was going to be said, he was quickly reassuring as he stated that his occupational therapist had been the most useful to him of anyone he had seen since his diagnosis of dementia. This gave me such a sense of pride in our profession to hear that occupational therapy had had a certain influence on his life. Little did I know at that point how positive both of them have been at embracing their life pre- and post-diagnosis, their involvement in research and their passion for activism to make a difference to individuals whose lives have been influenced by dementia.

I felt a great sense of responsibility when they evidently wanted me to tell their story in this chapter, and as time unfolded it has been a privilege spending time with them, hearing about their private world with the intention or focus of educating and inspiring others. To give some context, at the time of writing this chapter we were all experiencing the COVID-19 pandemic, which was having a significant impact on the occupations that all could engage in. Some examples of this may be evident in the stories shared, with both Chris and Jayne referring to a need to reintegrate with society over the coming months, and anticipating some challenges along the way.

From the outset of his diagnosis, Chris has been keen to learn as much as possible and to share his experiences to raise awareness of living positively with dementia. Chris and Jayne were clear that dementia was 'our diagnosis', as it impacted everyone in the family. This is evident throughout the chapter as examples are shared regarding their approach to daily life, of always looking for a solution and learning new skills. The conversations shared here over the course of several meetings online also highlight that both Chris and Jayne have become active members of several working groups related to dementia, locally, nationally and internationally.

'Pre-dementiaville and our road to a diagnosis'

Before they were married, Chris and Jayne had known each other for a long time and kept in touch through similar interests and friends. They met again later in life, married, and have children from previous relationships and two children together. Before receiving the diagnosis, dementia did not exist within their world. They had minimal awareness of dementia; it was no more than a word until this point, and then they said it 'hit us in the face'. At the beginning, Jayne and Chris were hit hard by the diagnosis, but after realizing Chris was still the same person, before diagnosis as after, 'we then picked ourselves up to get on with it'.

From spending time with Chris and Jayne, it is obvious that they enjoy spending time together and work together in a partnership. Following an accident, Jayne retired early on health grounds and has studied all over the world. They have shared bringing up the children, with

Chris working in a variety of roles including as a miner at the coalface, working in sales and developing his hobby of spraying motorbikes into a job. Chris also took on house maintenance for properties they rent out, choosing to learn practical skills. This role has continued and evolved with increasing support from Jayne since the diagnosis of dementia.

Early on, Chris discovered that a life-changing illness is just that: 'you have to change your life and that is what I have done'. Through researching dementia, it became an amazing help, and then, when they understood it, they chose to embrace it and live with it. Chris felt strongly that in the media, life-changing injuries or illnesses tend to be viewed so negatively, and 'yes, it can be, but people need to look for the positive changes'. For Chris and Jayne, this is when they looked at all problems as potential solutions, also acknowledging that there was a need to make adaptations in life.

Looking back, there were some early signs of cognitive changes that Chris and Jayne recalled. When completing an assessment with a 'young onset dementia' nurse, Jayne described Chris taking the bins out one night – he took them down into the village as he had forgotten to stop at the edge of their house. This highlighted that he could physically complete certain tasks, although at times, as a family, they needed to be mindful to provide Chris with prompts and instructions. Chris also ran his own motorbike shop that closed before his diagnosis, but on reflection, both can see some of the decisions he made were out of character and possibly related to the beginnings of dementia.

It was in 2012 that Chris and Jayne approached their doctor with concerns that led to a memory service referral. Following several visits, a mixed diagnosis of vascular dementia and Alzheimer's disease was given. Chris also has emphysema, which was diagnosed when he was in his forties.

'What do we need an occupational therapist for?'

From our first meeting back in 2018 it was obvious that Chris and Jayne had positive experiences from their contact with occupational therapists. Chris was initially referred to an occupational therapist for advice regarding falls. He was clear that he 'found the OT [occupational therapist] the master of everything', taking a helpful and practical approach. Jayne liked the 'Okay, what can *we* do about this?' approach.

The practical advice was valued as it pointed Chris and Jayne in the right direction, and encouraged them to get on with their life. Initially they were unsure of how an occupational therapist might help, but the more they understood the role of the occupational therapist, 'it sparked our minds, the adaptions we have made'. The occupational therapist gave 'light bulb moments' by suggesting that there were actually ways around things. This moved beyond the initial focus of 'what can't Chris do?'

From talking with Chris and Jayne there was a strong theme of problem-solving, keeping active, busy and learning new skills. All of these themes are key to occupational therapy, and below we have outlined some practical occupation-focused examples to highlight how Chris has adapted his daily life.

Transition from use of a computer to a tablet

Using a computer for emails, meetings and access to the internet is important to Chris. When he started having difficulty using the computer, his daughter introduced him to using a tablet, which was successful. Too much multitasking with the mouse, keyboard and separate screen was the challenge, and without switching to a tablet, Chris is clear: 'that would have been a skill lost'. Typing on a tablet also helped when writing became a challenge, as the keyboard comes up on the tablet, acting as a visual reminder of what letters look like. Using a tablet has moved on to Chris adding notes on how to complete tasks, such as making a cup of coffee.

Getting out and about

As Chris has chronic obstructive pulmonary disease (COPD), the occupational therapist facilitated a referral for a wheelchair. At the start, Jayne felt this was not linked to his dementia, but as Chris tired due to COPD, it would make his dementia worse, for example when out with the family shopping. Previously Chris would sit in cafes or on a bench, but in a lucid moment or when experiencing sensory overload, he would wander off. Chris was clear that the wheelchair 'made me feel very secure – a walled seat and my seat'.

The arrival of COVID-19 brought significant changes in lifestyle for all, and for Chris, he was 'happy in my bubble'. He kept busy in the garden, chopping things down, with Jayne accepting that plants 'will grow again'. Doing something purposeful is really important, although some people commented that Chris's involvement in conferences and training might be 'too much for him'. At times Chris would be involved in working groups and training others every week. Keeping different conversations going when at home has helped as it provides stimulation even though his cognition has deteriorated. Both Chris and Jayne describe concerns with re-engaging and reintegrating with society outside of the home or virtual world when restrictions are lifted following the pandemic, and people are no longer required to socially distance or be in lockdown at home.

Driving and work

Both Chris and Jayne are motorbike enthusiasts, so when Chris started having difficulties with manoeuvring the motorbikes, a conscious decision was made to sell their bikes: 'A tough decision to make and still have not got over it properly'. Jayne was concerned that Chris might forget one day, go out on a bike, and injure someone, so they decided to sell them. Chris described how the bikes felt different to handle on the road, which they now think was related to his balance. This was obviously not an easy decision as it also impacted on his work role and major occupation. A few years on, when Chris thought the motorbikes had been stolen, Jayne tried to soften the answer, but is clear that she never lies to Chris. She sensitively reminded him that the motorbikes had been sold and why.

Driving the work van to maintain properties also became an issue early on, and Chris thought he lived in a world of 'road rage where people were just beeping all of the time'. At this time, Chris was approaching 50 and was becoming less organized. He had previously had a very strong memory but started to not take the correct tools to complete a task in the rented house where he was working, and so he ended up travelling back and forth. His solution was to take all the tools in the van, which masked the changes in him for a while, but Jayne noted this difference. He also started taking different routes to properties, and so would make excuses for becoming disorientated in the local area.

Chris decided to surrender his driving licence after asking Jayne to observe him driving in the car. He was distracted and struggled with multitasking. Although Chris was aware he could have a driving test, he did not feel the need to take this as his wife had clearly pointed out that he was not safe driving, and he did not want to put people in danger. This was still not an easy decision, as having a driving licence is a 'rite of passage' and he felt that his independence and masculinity had 'gone overnight'. They had recently purchased a motorhome, so the timing was also difficult, but for Chris he describes that handing in his driving licence meant he felt empowered and that he was in charge, as 'I can still make decisions for myself even though I have got problems'.

At this point in terms of work, Jayne became the chauffeur and Chris made her the apprentice for house maintenance. Several years on, he still goes along to supervise and support her doing house maintenance, and often takes over the job and finishes it, as he can still do practical tasks with support.

Making a difference

From speaking with Chris and Jayne, the importance of making a difference through involvement in working groups, public speaking and informing policy was obviously key for both of them. For Chris, this stemmed from the public perception and stigma that often appears alongside a diagnosis of dementia, including phrases such as 'You don't look like you have dementia!' or 'Oh, you have dementia, but don't you look well!' Chris often uses the phrase 'You can't see my emphysema either', and this makes people think. Through hearing people's perceptions – not just the general public's, but also professionals' and academics' – Chris and Jayne have uncovered assumptions about people living with dementia that need to be challenged. This has led to them getting involved in local projects, Dementia Friends' education sessions and research.

Having to explain and justify what issues they were experiencing continually felt patronizing and also knocked Chris's confidence. It was interesting that through conversation it was felt that other hidden illnesses or disabilities could also be approached with the same thoughtlessness – 'if you can't see it, you haven't got it'. This led to a discussion around the terms 'hidden' or 'invisible' disability, with a preference for the term 'hidden' as dementia is not invisible and can be observed by others. Chris and Jayne wanted to highlight the value of using the sunflower lanyard to indicate a hidden disability when travelling by air. They feel this would act as a subtle visual cue to people who need to know in the airport or aircraft that he might require assistance. This has led to staff being more patient and speaking clearly, and Chris now uses this in supermarkets as well.

The following sections give a sense of the commitment and energy that Chris and Jayne bring as activists for promoting the rights of people living with dementia and their families. This is not an exhaustive list, but it will give an insight into how challenging assumptions can lead to positive change.

Local and national

From early on in their dementia journey, Chris chose to be a participant in dementia research. This has led to Jayne and Chris advising dementia research teams. They have been involved in writing books and co-authoring academic publications along with featuring in some television programmes.

As part of wanting to learn as much as they could about dementia and to share their experiences, Chris and Jayne were the first Dementia Friends in Wales, having completed their training session across the border in England. Being involved in providing Dementia Friends sessions as a Dementia Champion, Chris felt this gave him purpose. As people responded to him sharing his experiences, he realized he was challenging assumptions around what a person with dementia could and could not do. This was an important lesson as both Chris and Jayne realized the strength of presenting and then disclosing Chris had dementia towards the end of sessions. Their open approach has led to further public speaking, and they both realized this gave them the potential to change people's lives. Within a short space of time, they moved from delivering Dementia Friends sessions for a few local shops to presenting at the National Alzheimer's show and the Plaid Cymru (Party of Wales) conference. Receiving invitations to events helped them find out more about how to live with dementia, and it also gave them the chance to take information back to those who couldn't attend.

It was around this time that Jayne and Chris realized there was 'a whole machine around dementia' that involved networking, connecting people and getting involved with projects to improve people's lives. The role of connecting people is something Chris values, as he is aware that some introductions will help people. Involvement with DEEP (Dementia Engagement and Empowerment Project) in the UK has also been significant as it made a difference to Jayne and Chris hearing experiences and observing how this affected professionals in the audience. People presenting with dementia were treated as valued contributors, which further encouraged their involvement in sharing their experiences to educate others. This led to getting involved at government level with colleagues and the First Minister for Health in Wales launching 'Join Dementia Research', promoting and delivering talks to get people involved in dementia research and being ambassadors for the Alzheimer's Society. Chris is also a co-founder of the 3 Nations Dementia Working Group (3NDWG) (England, Northern Ireland and Wales), establishing their terms of reference, steering group and working relationship with the funders, the Alzheimer's Society.

Chris and Jayne have advocated for involvement of 'experts by experience' on Task and Finish and Steering Groups. They are clear that through being polite, reminding and educating people to give those with dementia respect, meaningful changes can be made to guidance and policy. A positive example of this was their involvement in the revision of the original Dementia Statements from the *National Dementia Declaration for England* (DAA 2010) in 2016/17. Originally, the statement began with 'I have, or I can...' with Chris insisting that the statements must be rights-based, and Jayne contributing the importance of changing 'I' to 'We', as all are in this together, including caregivers and professionals. Hence the Dementia Statements begin with 'We have the right...' The small group worked well together – 'you could feel it in the room – back and forth discussion and it worked'. The Dementia Action Alliance (DAA) adopted these statements across England (2017), and further rights-based documents have been developed across the UK.

Global

At the time of the conversations with Chris and Jayne, we were all restricted to staying at home in lockdown due to COVID-19. Their activist approach meant that they were still involved in regular international meetings across Europe and further afield online. They both highlight the importance of talking 'to the right people' who are 'interested in what he had to say about dementia'. This led to volunteering becoming a 'full-time job', and Chris describes that 'we were in a good place to be in a bad place – as we had time to go and do these things'.

This has led to roles on a European Working Group of People with Dementia, joining the Global Alzheimer's and DAA Group, and presenting in Australia and Japan. Chris described presenting in Japan to 5000 delegates as 'mind blowing' and an important educational role. Chris was also the first person to speak with dementia at a European patient involvement group.

When sharing their story, it was evident that becoming Salzburg Global Fellows in 2017 was a highlight for them both. Along with people from around the globe, the group met and created a statement regarding 'innovations in dementia care' and 'dementia-friendly communities' (Salzburg Global Seminar 2018). The Salzburg Global Seminar is a non-profit organization established to challenge current and future leaders to shape a better world.

In 2018, Chris was awarded a Bangor University Honorary Fellowship for 'Services to Research, Health and Social Care in Wales, the UK & Internationally' whilst serving as vice-chairperson of the European Working Group of People with Dementia (part of Alzheimer Europe), for whom he later became the chairperson. In 2019, Jayne received a Prime Minister's Point of Light award for being one of the UK's leading advocates for dementia. Receiving this award on St David's Day was a proud moment.

Closing remarks from Alison

It has been a privilege to spend time with Chris and Jayne to capture their story, which has been thought-provoking and inspiring – not only about their personal journey, but also about reinforcing the values of the occupational therapy profession, that through 'doing', people can be well. This chapter has highlighted some of the transition from diagnosis to then getting involved and becoming dementia activists. The need for training, awareness-raising and involving people with dementia from the outset of any work related to dementia is key. Chris and Jayne continue with their approach of always looking for a solution as involvement with voluntary work requires more support for Chris. They continue to be invested in wanting to make a positive difference to people living with dementia and their families through awareness-raising, education and generating debate.

Reflective questions

1. Identify key areas of occupation in which an occupational therapist has the potential to facilitate a person to continue to live their best with dementia.
2. What local policies and assessments are relevant for occupational therapists to gain an understanding of in relation to driving and dementia?
3. How can occupational therapists work collaboratively to promote the voice of people living with dementia?

References

DAA (Dementia Action Alliance) (2010) *National Dementia Declaration for England.* Accessed on 14/11/2021 at www.dementiaaction.org.uk

DAA (2017) *Review of the Dementia Statements: Companion Paper.* Accessed on 14/11/2021 at www.dementiaaction.org.uk/assets/0003/3965/Companion_document_August_2017_branded_final.pdf

Salzburg Global Seminar (2018) 'Salzburg global fellows call for innovations in dementia care and dementia-friendly communities.' Statements, 31 July. Accessed on 14/11/2021 at www.salzburgglobal.org/news/statements/article/salzburg-global-fellows-call-for-innovations-in-dementia-care-and-dementia-friendly-communities

CHAPTER 4

Occupational Therapy, Dementia and Person-Centredness

Brendan McCormack, Fiona Maclean and Lyn Westcott

Learning outcomes
By the end of this chapter, you will have the opportunity to:

▸ Understand the importance of personhood and the theory that informs the perspective of person-centred practice in care settings
▸ Reflect on person-centred cultures and ways of working that can enable all people to flourish
▸ Explore the ways through which personhood and person-centred ways of working can be integrated in occupational therapy practice for people living with dementia and their caregivers.

Introduction

In this chapter we explore person-centredness before moving on to contextualizing this to occupational therapy. We are, of course, all people, and occupational therapy focuses on enabling people to maximize their potential as citizens in society using occupation. Whilst we do not disagree with that fundamental position, 'person-centredness' is deeper and more complex in practice, embracing a myriad of complex philosophical, conceptual and theoretical perspectives. By exploring personhood as the underpinning philosophy of all person-centred working, we consider personhood for all, and the impact of different cultures on the way person-centred practices are realized. This has implications for the core principles and practices of occupational therapy, which are explored later in this chapter.

An overview of person-centredness

Contemporary health and social care is dominated by a discourse or language that emphasizes the virtues of people. This takes many shapes and forms, from extolling the virtues of individualized approaches to service provision, to the development of standards of practice that maximize the effectiveness of experience for people using services. Person-centredness embraces the multidimensions of people as the core focus of service delivery. It challenges politicians, organizations and care teams to focus on how best to meet the needs of individuals in context (Harding, Wait and Scrutton 2015; WHO 2016). At a superficial level, the term 'person-centred' is used to reflect the characteristics of high-quality health and social care, but a deeper understanding of person-centredness highlights its focus as humanizing services to ensure that the person living with dementia who uses these services is at the centre of decision-making.

Understanding and holding the values that are important to people using services and their families is the foundation of a person-centred approach to practice in dementia services and central to decision-making approaches. These values form the 'anchor' from which the quality of care is evaluated. This can, of course, create conflict as organizational and systems values may clash with those of individuals using services and families (Anjum *et al.* 2015). The skill involved in balancing a duty of care to people using services whilst also working with the 'best' evidence in decision-making is a significant challenge in person-centred dementia services (Miles and Asbridge 2013). Ensuring the person's identity is the central focus of decision-making, and helping to maintain the sense of who they are in the context of their lives, that is, their biography, is a key pillar of person-centred practice, and this is vital for people living with dementia.

Person-centred risk-taking is one of the biggest challenges that practitioners face in working in a person-centred way with people living with dementia. Practising in this way challenges health and social care practitioners to balance a commitment to evidence-based practice with, in our view, its focus on standardization, risk reduction and predetermined outcomes that can reinforce professional control over decision-making. Reducing the emphasis on professional control over care outcomes requires practitioners to work with choices that a person might make when their choices may be inconsistent with 'best evidence'. Thus, person-centredness requires professionals to balance professional and-personal knowledge as well as technical competence and expertise with the person's own choices, decisions, perceptions of their own wellbeing and their potential futures (van Dulmen *et al.* 2017). So, working in a person-centred way requires both personal courage and a practice culture that is committed to continuous, supportive, professional development.

Person-centred dementia practice makes explicit the need for auton-omy, equality and equity in relationships and the centrality of beliefs and values in guiding decision-making. For person-centred dementia practice to exist, there is a need for an organizational method that enables people to exercise power whilst simultaneously being able to negotiate how that power is exercised. This means we are obliged to build and sustain reflexive (that is, action informed by reflection) relationships, in working with others, whether colleagues or those referred to us. This practice also entails us making sense of others, and ourselves, as each of us creates conditions for growth, thriving and ways to personally flourish.

Taking all this into consideration, McCormack and McCance (2016, p.3) define person-centred practice as:

> an approach to practice established through the formation and fostering of healthful relationships between all care providers, service-users and others significant to them in their lives. It is underpinned by values of respect for persons, individual right to self-determination, mutual respect and understanding. It is enabled by cultures of empowerment that foster continuous approaches to practice development.

This definition of 'person-centred practice' makes explicit the values and beliefs that underpin such practices and the ways they are facili-tated. McCance and McCormack's person-centred practice framework (2021), which is derived from this definition, represents a whole-systems approach to the organizational development of person-centred services.

It pays attention to the macro (strategic and policy) context within which care is situated, as well as explicitly recognizing the qualities and attributes of practitioners needed to practice in person-centred ways. However, these qualities and attributes can only be realized if the context in which care workers practise is underpinned by a person-centred culture. This culture facilitates the realization of person-centred outcomes for all. There is an increasing body of evidence demonstrating the effectiveness of person-centred practices, and Phelan *et al.* (2020) synthesized this in a systematic literature review of global developments in person-centred healthcare. In this research five themes were highlighted that collectively demonstrate the global positioning of person-centredness in health and social care systems:

- Policy development for transformation
- Participatory strategies for public engagement
- Healthcare integration and coordination strategies
- Frameworks for practice
- Process and outcome measurement.

These themes reflect the World Health Organization (WHO) (2016) global perspective on people-centred and integrated systems, and identify development priorities as person-centred systems continue to develop and evolve. The review highlights the increased focus on person-centred developments that are underpinned by robust philosophical and theoretical frameworks, and that express clear values about 'the person' in person-centred care. The ways in which this literature has evolved is also important, as there has been an increasing emphasis on viewing person-centredness beyond the limited perspective of how people using services 'receive care' from providers, moving towards a perspective in which the whole culture of care needs to embrace person-centred values (McCormack *et al.* 2018). This shift in focus is an important one to emphasize, as without viewing person-centredness from a whole-systems culture perspective, the care received by people using services can never be guaranteed to be consistently person-centred. The development of cultures of person-centredness creates the capacity for all stakeholders (people using services, families and staff) to be viewed as 'people', and thus develop person-centred practice as an explicit shared purpose in organizations and teams.

Person-centred practice: being, knowing and becoming as people

Person-centred practice is underpinned by the philosophy of 'personhood', that is, the essence of being a person, articulated through complementary modes of 'being and becoming', that together enable all people to experience mutual respect and understanding (or sensing) in relationships. This concept is familiar to occupational scientists and occupational therapists through the work of Wilcock (1999) (see below), but is introduced here from the perspective of understanding person-centred practice. Personhood is not a static or fixed concept, and people are always in a state of becoming through reflective engagement, learning and transformation. Whilst personhood can be articulated through different philosophical traditions and concepts, we view it through the lens of five modes of being derived from the work of McCormack (2004) and Dewing (2004), whilst recognizing that people are always in a state of becoming:

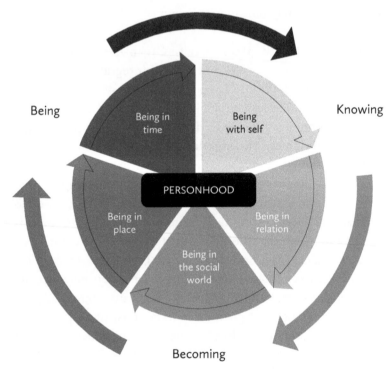

Figure 4.1. Knowing and becoming model

Being emphasizes the importance of relationships and the interpersonal processes that enable the development of relationships that benefit all people, enabling them to be 'the best that they can be'. People exist in context, and through that context we create and recreate meaning in our lives. Our context has a past, present and future, and as we grow and develop, we learn from this past to be present and authentic whilst looking to the future, all of which is informed by our core values that are continuously shaped by our context. People are connected in spaces and places that have physical, metaphysical and metaphorical meaning. Places connect people, and give meaning and shape to experience, as well as space for growth, development, comfort, nourishment, rejuvenation and stillness. People are temporal subjects and so 'time' is a dimension of our being and becoming as a person. Time is not a linear becoming made of instants. Instead, time flows through us whatever we do, enabling us to transition from the present, whilst allowing access to the past and future. For occupational therapists, the link between people and the notion of an enabling environment will be familiar and a precedent to using meaningful occupation. For those living with dementia, accessing the past through a present occupation allows a window to the essence of the person and their quality of life moving forward.

Respect for values is central to personhood, and these present a picture of what we privilege in life and how we make sense of different experiences. Knowing self through our core values provides a standard against which we compare current decisions and actions with those values and preferences made in life in general, and from which we form a life plan. People are simultaneously in a state of being and becoming. Through reflexive engagement with our five modes of being we come to know ourselves as both developed and developing people. Drawing on our embodied knowing and valued competencies we build our potential to envision an authentic future.

Mutuality is central to the process of collaborative relationships and decision-making, as it recognizes the equality of all people's values. A healthful relationship establishes a personal–professional connection based on mutual respect and understanding. It involves 'being with' and 'doing with', through active participation, the very essence of person-centred occupational therapy. Through mutual respect and understanding, people grow in each other's capacity to learn from each other as equals. As social beings, engagement is a way of working that reflects the connectedness of all people. If we accept that each situation is approached as a unique interaction, and that the focus is on the interaction with that person at that place and time, based on their values and beliefs, we can assume a collaborative approach to practice. The ability to engage and be truly connected with other people is dependent on our knowledge of the person, clarity of beliefs and values, knowledge of self and professional expertise. The existence of cultures that enable such engagement to happen and where all people can flourish is essential to person-centred practice.

Consider, for example, a cooking session in a day care facility, where people living with dementia work with staff to recreate a traditional local dish of rabbit pie. The reminiscences of needing to find cheap meat to feed the family and sharing experiences of how families ate with economy in mind illustrate how a unique interaction is collaborative and enables understanding of beliefs and values. Sharing an activity like this and the meaning it represents can help all people involved to understand one another, enhancing knowledge and connection.

Flourishing people, spaces and places

The term 'human flourishing' can be traced back to Aristotle who suggested that 'human flourishing occurs when a person is concurrently doing what he [sic] ought to do and doing what he wants to do'. This seemingly 'simple' definition of human flourishing is, in fact, highly complex and demanding of us. Aristotle positions our being as people in the world as moral frames, as an 'effective' person is one whose actions match those that people ought to have taken as a moral agent. When our actual and desired practices are interwoven, then we flourish as people. Of course, achieving this state requires that we operate in social and professional contexts that enable the integration of our being and doing as moral agents. Flourishing is not a project with a beginning or an end, and so creating workplaces and spaces that enable all people to flourish is a continuous and evolutionary process. No matter how much control we may feel over our lives, many internal and external influences, in terms of other people and our wider environment, shape us as well as the conditions that enable us to flourish as people (or not). Acknowledging this iterative cycle brings dynamism to practice and responds to the context and the people who shape that context and its ongoing transformation. McCormack and Titchen (2014, p.19) therefore suggest that flourishing is about energy and the flow of energy in and between people in connected relationships: 'Human flourishing occurs when we bound and frame naturally co-existing energies, when we embrace the known and yet to be known, when we embody contrasts and when we achieve stillness and harmony. When we flourish we give and receive loving kindness.'

Drawing on Buddhist philosophy, McCormack and Titchen (2014) suggest that when we are in connected and interconnected relationships and in contexts that are focused on enabling all people to flourish, we are receptive to giving and receiving 'loving kindness'. This focus on flourishing is consistent with McCormack and McCance's (2021) focus on the creating of healthful cultures as the ultimate outcome of person-centred practices. A healthful culture is one in which decision-making is shared, relationships are collaborative, leadership is transformational and innovative practices are supported, and is the ultimate outcome arising from the development of a workplace that enables human flourishing.

Occupational therapy and person-centred practice

The complexity and depth of person-centred practice highlighted so far relates, and has meaning, to the practice of occupational therapy when working with people living with dementia. Understanding person-centred practice in the context of working with people living with dementia, their families and caregivers is a key concept that offers an alternative, more hopeful approach than the historical adoption of the biomedical model (Bartlett and O'Connor 2010). Consequently, whilst it may seem obvious that occupational therapy practice aims to focus on enabling people living with dementia to maximize their potential as citizens in society, how and in what way the profession articulates this, influencing 'actions', is less clear.

An example may lie in the dichotomy of discourse that permeates our professional practice. Despite the growing recognition of the need for occupational therapists to be person-centred practitioners who underpin their practice with person-orientated principles and concepts (WFOT 2019), some of our theoretical conceptual models still consider client-centred practice rather than being person-centred in their approach. This is, for example, reflected in the Model of Human Occupation (MOHO)

(Taylor 2017) and the Canadian Model of Occupational Performance and Engagement (CMOP-e) (Townsend and Polatajko 2007). The tendency towards discussing client-centred practice is a point considered by Brown (2013), who suggests that the use of the term 'client' still suggests a power dynamic between people who use our services and practitioners. At a more specific level, the term 'client' also implies compartmentalization of therapy, which can challenge meeting the needs of people living with dementia. It implies something therapists do to people, as customers or consumers, rather than encouraging partnership. Working alongside people using collaborative approaches is fundamental to enabling people living with dementia to maintain and sustain independent lives for longer. This means as practitioners we need to consider both the language we use and what this suggests about how we work and what benefits people may gain from occupational therapy.

The term 'person-centred occupational practice', suggested by Brown (2013), may be a helpful step forward. This could be used to support occupational therapists and services committed to working with people living with dementia in valuing and retaining a focus on both occupation and person-centred working. In so doing, this extends attention beyond how people using services 'receive' care, but also more widely how occupational therapy teams create organizational cultures where all people can flourish. A key contributor to supporting a flourishing culture as occupational therapists is the ability of the profession to focus on how learning develops over time.

Consequently, how we approach and embrace ongoing learning and development is fundamental to how occupational therapists can seek to become person-centred practitioners. This need to accentuate learning and development that helps to promote and enact aspects of person-centred practice is noted by McCormack *et al.* (2021). Six elements of learning and development are explored as necessary to encourage person-centred practice. Some are broadly skills-based, like active learning and using reflection on the journey to knowing and becoming. Others mark the journey of the learner with a need for curiosity and research engagement including the mobilization of knowledge with practice. The learner journey continues as a lifelong commitment, drawing on critical thinking. The final element highlights the responsibility of the learner to develop and support others as practice educators, showing a movement of learning from the self to others.

A commitment to these elements throughout the career journey encourages a commitment to personal evolution. Or, to quote a phrase from Irvine, Gillen and Barr (2021, p.329), a 'growth mindset' can be nurtured. In so doing, this can help to fuel and inspire dynamism of person-centred occupational therapy in dementia services, acknowledging that both 'being' and 'becoming' for all, including people living with dementia and practitioners, can and does mean sharing a reciprocal opportunity to learn and grow from each other (see Chapter 10 in relation to reciprocity of learning).

Drawing on this perspective of personhood and underpinning theory, there is an obvious synergy with how the profession of occupational therapy understands the power of occupation, influencing health and wellbeing. The ideas of 'being' and 'becoming' in Figure 4.1, which flow into and inform our understanding of approaches to person-centred learning and development, are not unfamiliar to the profession. Wilcock (1999) has reflected on, and discussed, her seminal and influential contribution to how we as a profession think about occupation in terms of doing (occupation), being (nature and essence, being true to ourselves) and becoming (a sense of future, including transformation). It is beyond the scope of this chapter to untangle the similarity and differences that inevitably exist between these ideas from the perspectives of personhood (Dewing 2004; McCormack 2004) and occupation (Wilcock 1999). It is, however, worth acknowledging that a bond clearly exists, and requires further exploration and debate.

This offers a unique opportunity for occupational therapy to not only articulate a terminology of person-centred occupational practice, but importantly, to also give this shape and definition when working with people living with dementia, their families and caregivers. By taking time to engage with what might at first glance be an under-explored field of learning in our profession, person-centred practice, underpinned by the philosophy of 'personhood', as described in this chapter, offers an opportunity for the profession to grow. Specifically, when working with people living with dementia, their families and caregivers, the central focus of our professional contribution should be framed by a duality of approaches encompassing both the value and centrality of occupation, influenced and framed by person-centred cultures and a truly person-centred approach. In so doing, our ability to build healthful relationships for all people in the context of occupational therapy practice will help us to see the person, not their diagnosis of dementia, an aspiration encapsulated by a member of the Scottish Dementia Working Group (SDWG): 'I have dementia. It does not define me. My actions, hopes and dreams define me' (quoted in SDWG 2015).

Conclusion

This chapter has introduced the theory of personhood and person-centred practice in general terms. It has explored the key ideas guiding person-centred practice, highlighting the link between how people are in a constant state of being, knowing and becoming, and how practitioners can link in with this at a personal level to enhance meaningful care that understands the person's values and beliefs. It has highlighted some of the challenges at a wider level, including working with the person and the evidence that seeks to guide practice. The chapter has considered what person-centred practice means for occupational therapy, and how the approach challenges the notion of client-centred working in some occupational therapy models. It sets out a rationale for person-centred occupational therapy for people living with dementia and their families and caregivers. It suggests the six pillars put forward by McCormack *et al.* (2021) as a means to realize person-centred occupational therapy and the benefits this will bring.

Reflective questions

1. Watch a film, theatre production or narrative sharing experiences of people living with dementia. What key ideas in this chapter influence your understanding of that person's experience?

2. When reflecting on recent practice experience(s), in which contexts and in what ways have the terms 'client' and 'person' been used?

3. Choose one element of approaches to person-centred learning and development. Briefly summarize on a postcard how you have contributed to achieving this pillar over the last few months. Store the postcard somewhere safe and revisit it

in one year. What has changed in relation to your original thoughts, and how or why has this occurred?

References

Anjum, R.L., Copeland, S., Mumford, S. and Rocca, E. (2015) 'Integrating philosophical perspectives into person-centered healthcare.' *European Journal for Person Centered Healthcare 3*, 4, 427–430.

Bartlett, R. and O'Connor, D. (2010) *Broadening the Dementia Debate: Towards Social Citizenship*. Bristol: Policy Press.

Brown, T. (2013) 'Person-centred occupational therapy practice: Is it time for a change of terminology?' *British Journal of Occupational Therapy 76*, 5, 207.

Dewing, J. (2004) 'Concerns relating to the application of frameworks to promote person-centredness in nursing with older people.' *Journal of Clinical Nursing 13*, s1, 39–44.

Harding, E.W.S., Wait, S. and Scrutton, J. (2015) *The State of Play in Person-Centred Care: A Pragmatic Review of How Person-Centred Care Is Defined, Applied and Measured*. London: The Health Policy Partnership. Accessed on 22/04/2022 at www.healthpolicypartnership.com/app/uploads/The-state-of-play-in-person-centred-care.pdf

Irvine, L., Gillen, P. and Barr, O. (2021) 'Being a Lifelong Learner.' In B. McCormack, T. McCance, C. Bulley, D. Brown, A. McMillan and S. Martin (eds) *Fundamentals of Person-Centred Healthcare Practice* (pp.319–330). Oxford: Wiley Blackwell.

McCance, T. and McCormack, B. (2021) 'The Person-Centred Practice Framework.' In B. McCormack, T. McCance, C. Bulley, D. Brown, A. McMillan and S. Martin (eds) *Fundamentals of Person-Centred Healthcare Practice* (pp.23–32). Oxford: Wiley Blackwell.

McCormack, B. (2004) 'Person-centredness in gerontological nursing: An overview of the literature.' *Journal of Clinical Nursing 13*, s1, 31–38.

McCormack, B. and McCance, T. (2016) *Person-Centred Practice in Nursing and Health-care: Theory and Practice*. Oxford: Wiley Blackwell.

McCormack, B. and Titchen, A. (2014) 'No beginning, no end: An ecology of human flourishing.' *International Practice Development Journal 4*, 2. Accessed on 22/04/2022 at www.fons.org/library/journal/volume4-issue2/article2

McCormack, B., Dickson, C., Smith, T., Ford, H., *et al.* (2018) '"It's a nice place, a nice place to be". The story of a practice development programme to further develop person-centred cultures in palliative and end of life care.' *International Practice Development Journal 8*, 1. Accessed on 22/04/2022 at https://doi.org/10.19043/ipdj81.002

McCormack, B., McCance, T., Bulley, C., Brown, D., McMillan, A. and Martin, S. (2021) *Fundamentals of Person-Centred Healthcare Practice*. Oxford: Wiley Blackwell.

Miles, A. and Asbridge, J.E. (2013) 'Contextualizing science in the aftermath of the evidence-based medicine era: On the need for person-centred health care.' *European Journal for Person Centered Health Care 1*, 2, 285–289.

Phelan, A., McCormack, B., Dewing, J., Brown, D., *et al.* (2020) 'Review of developments in person-centred healthcare.' *International Practice Development Journal 10*, 2. Accessed on 22/04/2022 at http://doi.org/10.19043/ipdj.10Suppl2.003

SDWG (Scottish Dementia Working Group) (2015) 'This is me – Henry Rankin.' Edinburgh: SDWG. Accessed on 19/10/2021 at www.youtube.com/watch?v=xDM7Nd7yBSA

Taylor, R. (2017) *Kielhofner's Model of Human Occupation* (5th edn). Philadelphia, PA: Wolters Kluwer.

Townsend, E. and Polatajko, H. (2007) *Enabling Occupation II: Advancing an Occupational Therapy Vision for Health, Well-Being and Justice Through Occupation*. Ottawa, ON: CAOT Publications ACE.

van Dulmen, S., McCormack, B., Eide, H., Eide, T. and Skovdal, K. (2017) 'Future Directions for Person-Centred Research.' In B. McCormack, S. van Dulman, H. Eide, K. Skovdahl and T. Eide (eds) *Person-Centred Healthcare Research* (Chapter 18). Oxford: Wiley & Sons.

WFOT (World Federation of Occupational Therapists) (2019) *Occupational Therapy and Community-Centred Practice*. Position Statement. London: WFOT. Accessed on 19/10/2021 at www.wfot.org/resources/occupational-therapy-and-community-centred-practice

WHO (World Health Organization) (2016) *Framework on Integrated, People-Centred Health Services*. Geneva: WHO. Accessed on 19/10/2021 at https://apps.who.int/gb/ebwha/pdf_files/WHA69/A69_39-en.pdf?ua=1

Wilcock, A.A. (1999) 'Reflections on doing, being and becoming.' *Australian Journal of Occupational Therapy 46*, 1, 1–11.

CHAPTER 5

The Role of Occupational Therapy in Promoting Lifelong Brain Health

Neil Fullerton, Fiona Maclean, Elaine Hunter and Anna Borthwick

Learning outcomes

By the end of this chapter, you will have the opportunity to:

▸ Understand the evolution of diseases that cause dementia across the lifespan, which has propelled a shift in focus towards brain health and prevention
▸ Be able to identify and describe the modifiable risk factors that can influence a person's risk of developing dementia
▸ Explore the potential contribution of occupational therapy to dementia prevention and public health messaging across the lifespan.

Introduction

Increasingly there is a call to occupational therapists to consider how and in what way their work can contribute to public and population health. Whilst various definitions of public and population health exist, for the purposes of this chapter, these terms are defined as, 'the science and art of promoting and protecting health and wellbeing, preventing ill health and prolonging life through the organised efforts of society' (Hindle and Charlesworth 2019, p.7).

Preventing dementia is a global responsibility (Alzheimer's Disease

International 2019). This has influenced a commitment and response from the Scottish Government, who have worked in partnership with Scotland's leading dementia charity, Alzheimer Scotland, to develop and advance wider appreciation of the need to understand the importance of population brain health across the lifespan.

This chapter therefore begins by presenting the science and research that underpins ongoing and evolving work that informs the current state of knowledge in brain health. By extension, this offers an opportunity to explore how, and in what way, professional knowledge of brain health, that is, maintaining a healthy brain, can influence the role of occupational therapy in public and population health promotion. Consequently, the chapter concludes by examining the window of opportunity that exists for the profession to begin to work with asymptomatic, yet at-risk, groups of people, before a diagnosis of dementia, as part of communities and across populations, to begin to define and promote the health-giving power of occupation to dementia prevention.

Context and background to promoting brain health

Over recent decades research has given us a much greater understanding of the natural history of diseases that lead to dementia. The term 'dementia' is an umbrella term, used to define a clinical syndrome where diseases of the brain have advanced to such a stage that they cause overt cognitive symptoms and functional impairment. The majority of cases of dementia are the result of neurodegenerative disease processes. Neurodegenerative diseases are progressive life-limiting diseases of the central nervous system that are caused by dysfunction, degradation, and ultimately, the death of neurons (brain cells). The most common of these conditions is Alzheimer's disease.

The pathological processes that cause brain cells to die, and ultimately lead to symptoms, build up slowly over time. As such, they have a long asymptomatic or clinically silent period that stretches back many years before obvious cognitive symptoms and functional difficulties become apparent (see Figure 5.1). Alzheimer's disease biomarkers, which are bodily characteristics that can be measured to indicate the state of health or disease, are known to become abnormal 15–25 years prior to the onset of a dementia syndrome (Villemagne *et al.* 2013). So, whilst symptom onset most commonly, though not exclusively, occurs over the age of 65, the origins of disease are grounded firmly within the age range of mid-life. As such, focusing solely on the dementia phase of illness is to focus only on later-stage disease.

This has propelled a recent shift to considering brain health across the life course, rather than focusing solely on the symptomatic stage of disease. This informs the need to consider key public health messages that need to be disseminated at a population level as well as particular attention required to engage at-risk groups. The updated model of engaging asymptomatic, at-risk individuals brings a shift in focus of the healthcare workforce traditionally considered to operate in the dementia space, emphasizing the need for the profession of occupational therapy to understand the relevance and possibilities of professional contribution to neurodegenerative disease prevention.

Opportunities for prevention

The long clinically silent period of these diseases, stretching back many years before the onset of dementia, offers a substantial window of opportunity to intervene in the pre-symptomatic stages to significantly delay or even prevent progression to symptomatic disease. With a progressive disease course that builds in severity slowly over time, it is possible to consider three distinct time frames in which to implement prevention strategies (see Figure 5.1).

- Primary prevention: Acting before a disease is present to ensure a person never develops that condition.
- Secondary prevention: Intervening in the early stages of disease, where disease processes have begun, but not yet progressed in severity to cause symptoms.
- Tertiary prevention: Managing a disease in the symptomatic phase, with the aim of limiting the impact, minimizing disability and maximizing quality of life.

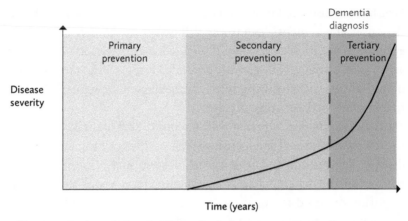

Figure 5.1. Brain pathology builds up slowly for many years preceding symptom onset and a dementia diagnosis, providing windows of opportunity for prevention

Until now, treatment and care for neurodegenerative diseases has focused almost exclusively on tertiary prevention, at the stage following a dementia diagnosis. This is in part because it has been very difficult to identify people and intervene in this secondary prevention window when, by definition, there are no symptoms to pick up on.

The situation is changing, as large and in-depth longitudinal research studies are providing a much more detailed understanding of the pre-symptomatic stage of disease (Mueller *et al.* 2005; Ritchie *et al.* 2016; Sperling *et al.* 2020). In particular, these studies have driven forwards knowledge of specific biomarkers, which mean people can be identified at a much earlier stage of disease.

This will not only serve to improve scientific understanding, but crucially, it is also going to shift the way conditions like Alzheimer's disease are diagnosed, managed and lived with, which will fundamentally broaden the nature and scope of professional contribution, including occupational therapy practice. This understanding means that occupational therapists will need to begin to include and refocus elements of their practice to work in partnership with those living with a diagnosis of early-stage neurodegenerative disease, rather than the initial diagnosis being one of dementia.

People living with early-stage neurodegenerative disease will need support adjusting to a long-term progressive condition at, on average, a much earlier stage of life than most current dementia-focused services are designed for. This is likely to mean therapists will need to acquire wider knowledge and understanding of designing and implementing a range of self-management techniques and interventions, which will encompass both practical and emotional support. The potential contribution of the profession of occupational therapy in this regard is considered in more detail later in this chapter. Suffice to say here, the occupational therapists of today, tomorrow and the future must begin to prepare now for this major shift in what people will know about their own brain health. They must be proactive in helping individuals manage the way forward, living with neurodegenerative disease, whilst in tandem continuing to offer the best possible standard of care for those people living with dementia.

Towards risk profiling

As the focus on early detection of disease becomes stronger, secondary prevention strategies will dominate clinical management for this population. Ideally, however, it is always preferable to target primary prevention, to stay well and build resilience, rather than react to disease once it has developed.

To most effectively focus and prioritize both primary and secondary prevention initiatives, it is important to determine an individual's risk status for developing neurodegenerative disease. Understanding of the various factors that contribute towards disease risk has grown enormously over recent decades. Now is the time to translate this knowledge to successfully inform strategies that promote brain health.

Modifiable risk factors

Areas of risk for developing a particular disease can be divided into two broad categories: fixed risk factors and modifiable risk factors. Fixed risks are those things we cannot do anything about, whereas modifiable risks have at least the potential to be addressed or reduced.

When considering the diseases that can lead to dementia, there are fixed risk factors, such as age and genetics, that have a major influence on the likelihood of developing the condition (Pihlstrøm, Wiethoff and Houlden 2018). However, there are also many modifiable risk factors that contribute towards the overall balance of risk, and which can, through lifestyle, behavioural and societal changes, be effectively managed.

All occupational therapists have a role to play in promoting prevention (Council of Deans 2021) and therefore in being aware of these potentially manageable risk factors, many of which are already commonly understood in the context of other areas of health, such as cardiovascular health and cancer risk. Links to neurodegenerative disease, however, are less well known, and it is this association that must be communicated effectively from healthcare professionals to the people they support.

The individual risk factors for which we have the greatest level of evidence to date are collated in the Lancet Commission report on dementia prevention, intervention and care (Livingston *et al.* 2020). This report concludes that eliminating 12 potentially modifiable factors on a population-wide level would lead to a projected 40 per cent decrease in the total number of cases of all-cause dementia worldwide (see Table 5.1).

Table 5.1. Modifiable risk factors for the development of dementia

Life stage	Risk factor for dementia
Early life	1. Less education
Mid life	2. Hearing loss
	3. Traumatic brain injury
	4. Hypertension
	5. Alcohol (>21 units/week)
	6. Obesity
Later life	7. Smoking
	8. Depression
	9. Social isolation
	10. Lack of physical activity
	11. Air pollution
	12. Type 2 diabetes

Source: Adapted from Livingston et al. (2020)

This comprehensive report only includes factors with substantial, high-quality current evidence. Emerging evidence is growing all the time around the importance of several other factors, such as sleep and the role of stress, to name just two. Through increased research interest in this area, understanding will continue to be broadened, ultimately providing a greater range of interventional strategies.

The headline figure of 40 per cent of cases being, in theory, preventable represents population-wide calculations largely based on data from high-income countries. In practice, no plan of action, no matter how ambitious in scope, could be successful in eliminating these factors entirely from the global population. It is also clear that many of the risk factors listed have complex aetiologies and interrelated associations themselves. However, the factors identified do provide a valuable insight into key areas on which to focus attention and concentrate prevention initiatives.

A life course approach

Symptom onset may be most commonly associated with later life; however, there are clearly many opportunities to act throughout life to help protect and maintain brain structure and function and reduce the risk of later life disease. As risks to brain health accumulate throughout life, there are important protective steps to be considered right from early life education, through to critical periods in mid life, through to later-life cognitive and social stimulation.

Importantly, framing lifelong action in this way facilitates a proactive and empowering approach to brain health, reinforcing that there are positive steps that everyone can make to take a certain degree of ownership over improving their brain health.

There remains, across many populations, a false perception of dementia as an inevitable consequence of ageing. Surprisingly, this opinion is also highly pervasive amongst health professional groups, as highlighted by the Alzheimer's Disease International 'Attitudes to Dementia Survey' that reported almost two-thirds of healthcare practitioners thought that dementia is a normal part of ageing (Alzheimer's Disease International 2019). It is clear, therefore, that not enough has been done to effectively disseminate updated knowledge, and a lack of relevant awareness persists.

Studies of post-mortem brain tissue have consistently shown that not all individuals are affected equally by the presence of neurodegenerative processes. Two people who demonstrate the same degree of pathology in the brain can have extremely different presentations in terms of the severity of symptoms and functional impairment they experience in life (Negash *et al.* 2013).

The precise mechanisms underlying this variation in symptom

presentation is not definitively known. However, one prominent theory for why this may be is explained through the concept of 'cognitive reserve' (Stern 2012). The model of cognitive reserve posits that if an individual has a richer network of pathways built up in their brain, through a greater number of interlinked brain cell connections (synapses), they may then be able to tolerate a larger degree of brain damage before experiencing detrimental symptoms. In theory, this richer developed network of connections makes an individual more resilient, more able to re-route, adapt or compensate when damage occurs and, ultimately, to tolerate early brain disease processes.

Regardless of the precise biological and compensatory mechanisms underlying these observed variations, the general principle reinforces the importance of incorporating brain health messaging from early years education onwards, and that continuing these constructive practices at all stages of life will benefit individuals spanning the entire spectrum of risk. This messaging should be positive and promote an approach that builds brain resilience to significantly delay, or even prevent altogether, the onset of symptoms.

The evidence presented in the Lancet Commission report (Livingston *et al.* 2020) emphasized that there are common, broad-brush stroke approaches that can be made to benefit large proportions of the population, and that doing so can have a significant impact on population-level incidence of symptomatic disease. These approaches, emerging from the science and research presented here, can therefore be used as the basis to inform public health interventions and the contribution of occupational therapy.

The health-giving power of occupation to brain health

Other chapters in this book directly address the contribution of occupational therapy with people living with dementia, their families and caregivers. Here, the context of professional commitment is to emphasize the rights of people across their life course to access occupational engagement to enhance their health and wellbeing.

Occupational therapists typically work alongside people across a range of practice settings, often because of the comorbidities described in Table 5.1. Irrespective of practice speciality, promoting occupational engagement will influence a person's wellbeing and promote brain health not only at the point of contact, but also into the future. The right to access occupation therefore plays a crucial role in reducing risk for the future development of dementia, and therapists across the profession should understand this general health-promoting message.

However, it is also necessary to widen the potential scope of professional contribution to health promotion beyond existing practice settings. New approaches are needed to sustain health and wellbeing across our communities, and increasingly the allied health professions, including occupational therapy, are seen as essential to this revised approach (Council of Deans 2021; Hindle and Charlesworth 2019). Professions such as occupational therapy can refocus support, designed to provide the optimal conditions with which to proactively maintain brain health throughout life, thus building resilience and helping prevent disease onset from occurring. For example, the profession will have an important role to play in facilitating primary prevention initiatives through developing and extending their focus on public and population health.

Modifiable risk factors that could influence the health of an individual's brain, including those listed in Table 5.1, could be positively addressed through six key areas of action. Each of these potential areas of public health interventions, listed below (adapted from Brain Health Scotland 2021), could be led by occupational therapists:

- *Creativity:* Occupational therapy is a profession that has emerged from an understanding of the benefits to health and wellbeing of creativity because learning new skills throughout life can help keep the brain stimulated and build resilience. Our profession provides diverse examples of how we can use creativity in practice, from poetry to gaming, from painting to animation. The right to new and creative occupations available as part of local communities should be encouraged across the life course, and led by occupational therapists.
- *Social connection:* Regular and fulfilling social interaction is crucially important to reducing social isolation and maintaining brain health. As occupational therapists we have knowledge and understanding of the need to bring people together – collective occupation – in a setting people enjoy, providing an opportunity to be creative and to stay active.

- *Rest:* An important contributor to good sleep (7–9 hours for adults), reducing stress is vital to maintaining brain health. Occupational therapists are able to offer practical advice on good sleep hygiene, and effective, tailored methods for managing stress and evidence-based advice on looking after mental health.
- *Activity:* Regular exercise that raises the heart rate and reduces sedentary behaviour is essential for good brain health. Occupational therapists help people to maintain activity that is important to them. By setting personalized goals with people, based on an understanding of what matters to them, the profession values and prompts diversity of activity – for example, dancing at a wedding, walking to the local shop or continuing to play bowls.
- *Healthy eating:* Eating a Mediterranean-style diet that promotes cardiovascular health is important to brain health. This wider health-promoting message is a core responsibility of all health practitioners, including occupational therapists, to support behavioural change throughout the life course in relation to healthy eating.
- *Smoking and drinking:* It is important to avoid smoking and drinking to excess. Occupational therapy research exploring drinking as an occupation in later life (Maclean *et al.* 2020) seeks to promote wider professional awareness of alcohol consumption in older age.

The concept of continuing cognitive and social engagement as crucial to brain health at all stages of life is of particular significance to the profession. For example, the value of people 'coming together' can be understood through the lens of collective occupation (Kantartzis and Molineux, 2017) – that is, occupations undertaken in groups, with friends, as part of local communities, which can support and nurture happier and healthier relationships.

In addition, these six areas of public health interventions offer a starting point to address the practice of occupational therapy in relation to population brain health. Yet, these must be set within the context of an understanding of those who are most likely to be excluded from opportunities to stay socially connected or get creative. In the UK this need is pressing. Whilst life expectancy in other European countries continues to improve, in the UK it has stalled, in part due to health inequalities (Marmot 2019). Targeted population health interventions should therefore acknowledge occupation as a human right and a core element of practice, particularly for those who live in poverty and in areas of deprivation. Equality of reach and of access to brain health guidance and services should be central to inclusive care.

Moreover, a move towards promoting preventative measures for dementia across the entire life course mediates a shift in the population typically targeted for engagement and intervention. Engaging groups and individuals with a higher risk profile will necessarily involve input from occupational therapists who work with children and young people, as well as therapists working in public health, primary care or hospital and community settings. Approaches will need to be identified that can reach these at-risk groups for whom the concept of brain health and pre-clinical disease phases may well be new information, groups who understandably may not self-identify as harbouring risk factors for brain disease.

As such, an open-minded approach should be adopted as to where these groups may come into contact with occupational therapy services. As the demographic of who benefits from effective risk reduction strategies widens, these groups and individuals will not exclusively be found within traditional dementia-focused healthcare services. High levels of collaboration between occupational therapists and other health and social care services will be essential to enable effective and inclusive care.

Conclusion

To complement public health approaches, occupational therapists can use an increased understanding of risk factors, coupled with a greater ability to detect disease early through biomarker analysis, to take more of a precision approach, customized for an individual, the ultimate aim being to develop personalized prevention plans, informed by:

- Detailed risk profiling
- Early detection of disease where present
- Tailored interventions that address risk factors to reduce an individual's likelihood of disease progression.

A major area of focus for such prevention plans will be on interventions promoting independence, wellbeing and social engagement to help an individual stay connected. This suggests that the profession of occupational therapy has a significant role to play in promoting public health by encouraging brain health in the future. However, whilst the relationship between the profession of occupational therapy and the aims of public health promotion have frequently been highlighted as important in professional literature, practice does not often reflect this goal (Hocking 2011). In part this may be due to the paucity of educational content addressing health promotion and wellness approaches in entry-level programmes (Morris and Jenkins 2018). However, one example of where this educational gap is beginning to be addressed in the UK is that the Royal College of Occupational Therapists (RCOT) (2019) pre-registration (entry-level) learning and development standards for professional programmes must now include public health and prevention concepts.

As such, this chapter offers an important contribution in helping to define how occupational therapy can begin to orchestrate evidence-based public health and wellbeing approaches to help prevent neurodegenerative disease and dementia. This will include occupational therapists acting as a primary healthcare contact for an individual, overseeing the establishment and ongoing management of personalized prevention plans. In addition, the context of practice will include working with communities, where the foundation of approaches adopted will emerge from an understanding of the value of relationships and occupation tailored to the person, their risk factors, and for the benefit of their brain health.

Reflective questions

1. Consider the three distinct time frames that exist to implement disease prevention strategies (primary, secondary and tertiary). How, and in what way, might you design occupation-focused health and wellbeing approaches to help prevent neurodegenerative disease?
2. With a focus on social connection and relationships, how, and in what way, might you translate ideas connected to collective occupation(s) in designing health promotion and wellbeing

approaches with your community? For example, your community could be family and friends, your university and occupational therapy learners, etc.

3. What would you include in a newspaper article or opinion piece to highlight the role of occupational therapy in promoting brain health?

References

Alzheimer's Disease International (2019) *World Alzheimer Report 2019: Attitudes to Dementia*. London: Alzheimer's Disease International. Accessed on 01/11/2021 at www.alzint.org/resource/world-alzheimer-report-2019

Brain Health Scotland (2021) *Your Brain Is Amazing: Let's Keep It That Way*. Edinburgh: Brain Health Scotland. Accessed on 30/10/2021 at www.brainhealth.scot

Council of Deans (2021) *Guidance: Public Health Content within the Pre-Registration Curricula for Allied Health Professions*. London: Council of Deans of Health.

Hindle, L. and Charlesworth, L. (2019) *UK Allied Health Professions Public Health Strategic Framework: 2019–2024*. AHPF (Allied Health Professions Federation). Accessed on 30/10/2021 at www.health-ni.gov.uk/sites/default/files/publications/health/uk-ahp-public-health.pdf

Hocking, C. (2011) 'Public Health and Health Promotion.' In L. Mackenzie and G. O'Toole (eds) *Occupation Analysis in Practice* (pp.246–263). Chichester: Wiley-Blackwell.

Kantartzis, S. and Molineux, M. (2017) 'Collective occupation in public spaces and the construction of the social fabric.' *Canadian Journal of Occupational Therapy 84*, 168–177.

Livingston, G., Huntley, J., Sommerlad, A., Ames, D., *et al.* (2020) 'Dementia prevention, intervention, and care: 2020 report of the Lancet Commission.' *The Lancet 396*, 10248, 413–446.

Maclean, F., Dewing, J., Kantartzis, S., Breckenridge, J.P., *et al.* (2020) 'Can we talk about it? A qualitative study exploring occupational therapists' decision making in judging when to ask an older person about drinking alcohol.' *Ageing & Society*. Accessed on 22/04/2022 at https://doi.org/10.1017/S0144686X20000951

Marmot, M. (2019) 'There can be no more important task than to reduce health inequalities.' The Health Foundation Blog, 27 February. Accessed on 30/10/2021 at www.health.org.uk/news-and-comment/blogs/there-can-be-no-more-important-task-than-to-reduce-health-inequalities

Morris, D.M. and Jenkins, G.R. (2018) 'Preparing physical and occupational therapists to be health promotion practitioners: A call for action.' *International Journal of Environmental Research and Public Health 15*, 392, 1–12.

Mueller, S.G., Weiner, M.W., Thal, L.J., Petersen, R.C., *et al.* (2005) 'Ways toward an early diagnosis in Alzheimer's disease: The Alzheimer's Disease Neuroimaging Initiative (ADNI).' *Alzheimer's & Dementia 1*, 1, 55–66.

Negash, S., Wilson, R.S., Leurgans, S.E., Wolk, D.A., *et al.* (2013). 'Resilient brain aging: Characterization of discordance between Alzheimer's disease pathology and cognition.' *Current Alzheimer Research 10*, 8, 844–851.

Pihlstrøm, L., Wiethoff, S. and Houlden, H. (2018) 'Genetics of neurodegenerative diseases: An overview.' *Handbook of Clinical Neurology 145*, 309–323.

RCOT (Royal College of Occupational Therapists) (2019) *Learning and Development Standards for Pre-Registration Education.* London: RCOT. Accessed on 30/10/2021 at www.rcot.co.uk/practice-resources/rcot-publications/learning-and-development-standards-pre-registration-education

Ritchie, C.W., Molinuevo, J.L., Truyen, L., Satlin, A., *et al.* (2016) 'Development of interventions for the secondary prevention of Alzheimer's dementia: The European Prevention of Alzheimer's Dementia (EPAD) project.' *The Lancet Psychiatry 3*, 2, 179–186.

Sperling, R.A., Donohue, M.C., Raman, R., Sun, C.K., *et al.* (2020) 'Association of factors with elevated amyloid burden in clinically normal older individuals.' *JAMA Neurology 77*, 6, 735–745.

Stern, Y. (2012) 'Cognitive reserve in ageing and Alzheimer's disease.' *The Lancet Neurology 11*, 11, 1006–1012.

Villemagne, V.L., Burnham, S., Bourgeat, P., Brown, B., *et al.* (2013) 'Amyloid β deposition, neurodegeneration, and cognitive decline in sporadic Alzheimer's disease: A prospective cohort study.' *The Lancet Neurology 12*, 4, 357–367.

ENVIRONMENT

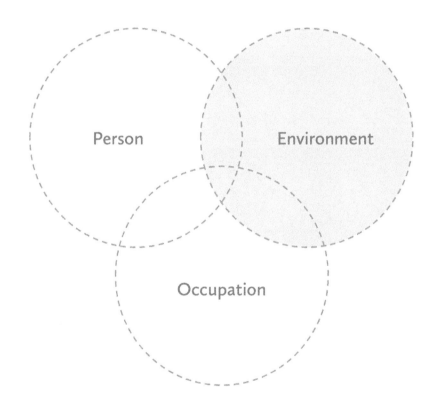

CHAPTER 6

People with Dementia and Social Transformation

Expanding Occupational Possibilities

Sarah Kantartzis, Debbie Laliberte Rudman and Fiona Maclean

Learning outcomes

By the end of this chapter, you will have the opportunity to:

▶ Consider people as citizens embedded in networks of relationships and occupations at the core of occupational therapy practice

▶ Explore the way social structures, including discourses, and practices shape the everyday lives of people with dementia

▶ Explore how age and its intersection with dementia can be framed as axes of diversity, or markers of social difference, that influence occupational possibilities

▶ Develop knowledge of the concept and processes of social transformation through occupation, through practice examples linked to effecting change to improve the lives of people with dementia.

Introduction

As social animals, people are interconnected and engaged in constructing their social world together through occupation. Our daily lives and our shared occupations as citizens are shaped not only by our personal preferences and abilities but also by historical, cultural, economic and political factors (Pollard *et al.* 2021). Discourses, that is, how a social issue or group is written and talked about, are shaped by such factors and come to influence everyday possibilities for occupation (Laliberte Rudman 2006).

This chapter will focus in particular on the power of discourses to shape the value given to various groups of people and the possibilities for occupation available to them. One example will be discussed, that of age, to demonstrate how power relations construct markers of diversity in ways that bound occupational possibilities. In a similar manner, and intersecting with social markers such as age or gender, diagnoses can also be viewed as an axis of difference or diversity that can further shape what we come to see as the 'right', ideal and healthy occupations for particular groups, including people living with dementia, as well as what come to be viewed as the 'wrong', non-ideal and impossible occupations for them. These taken-for-granted constructions of occupational possibilities are, in turn, embedded in practices, including occupational therapy practices, institutional policies and various forms of media, thereby influencing which occupations are supported, when and how.

Occupation-based social transformation recognizes the power of occupation to effect change not only in the everyday lives of individuals but also at broader societal levels – change in social practices, systems and structures including discourses, to improve the lives of particular groups of people, particularly those at risk of exclusion or marginalization (van Bruggen *et al.* 2020). In the case of people living with dementia, these ideas help to recognize the need to look beyond the individual, to consider wider, often unnoticed influencers of exclusion, such as socioeconomic status, as well as discursive representations and how these can impact how and in what way people living with dementia can experience stigma and associated marginalization from the everyday life of their communities.

A focus on occupation-based social transformation offers a wider perspective to understand how and in what way often-unintentional boundaries can shape the occupational possibilities of those living with dementia. Crucially, it also offers an opportunity to respond. Concluding this chapter, we illustrate this with an example of a project that adopted the use of photography to counter the often taken-for-granted assumptions connected to the occupational possibilities of people living with dementia, including what seem to be some of the key characteristics of the processes of such initiatives.

Considering citizenship and occupation in the public world

Humans are social animals, living in groups and arranging their lives together. How we live together has been organized through a range of formal and informal rules and regulations over time. Core to these processes is the idea of citizenship, that in living together we take on rights and responsibilities not only with the state, but also between each other. Whilst globally there are numerous forms of citizenship, including those primarily focused on the legal status of 'citizenship' of a particular nation, they also include much broader ideas. These recognize the importance of how we live together, with a right to discuss, debate, participate and take action in all things that affect our everyday lives, as we recognize each other as equals, with dignity and respect for our diversity (Hoskins *et al.* 2012; Pollard *et al.* 2021).

This right to be part of the public world involves our participation in collective occupations (Kantartzis and Molineux 2017). The idea of collective occupation raises awareness of the importance of our daily lives with others, our essential interrelatedness, and how the practice of our daily lives is shaped and shapes the social fabric that we are all part of. Many of our daily occupations we do with, for or because of other people. These include those informal encounters with other people as we go shopping or just walk down our street – the smile, the hand-shake, the greeting and enquiry of how we are support us to feel part of 'our' neighbourhood or town, and happen because we are aware of each other and acknowledge that we share these everyday spaces. Other occupations are opportunities to share the excitement of the football match, the relaxation of the pub and the game of darts, the joy of singing together or to share memories at a family memorial. Such occupations help to shape and express our emotions as well as feel connected with others. Different, again, are those collective occupations that call on our skills and our passions as we work with others around issues of common interests, perhaps advocating for local issues, arranging a street party or volunteering in the local food bank (Kantartzis and Molineux 2017). In such multiple ways we engage as citizens, we practise citizenship, in our shared public world.

Citizenship is increasingly viewed as important in discussions to understand dementia. The practice of citizenship emphasizes the essential interrelationship of people with dementia with their communities (Bartlett and O'Connor 2010), as political citizens with rights as well as agency (O'Connor and Nedlund 2016). However, the concept is also important due to its essential incorporation of ideas of the power of sociocultural practices and assumptions, which traditionally have placed people with dementia as less able or less worthy (O'Conner and Nedlund 2016). Collective occupation may put into practice such beliefs and perceptions, restricting people's opportunities to engage in certain occupations.

Considering occupational possibilities

Supporting citizenship and doing in the public world has been increasingly framed as central in occupational therapy. As one example – the 2021 World Federation of Occupational Therapists' (WFOT) Position Statement addressing ageing across the life course highlights the role and responsibility of occupational therapists to 'promote the rights and opportunities for older adults to engage in occupations of choice and need' (2021, p.1).

This highlights the importance of enacting a rights-based approach through occupational therapy to ensure all citizens, across the life course, have possibilities to engage in desired occupations and be part of the social fabric of communities. Given that what people can and cannot do is always shaped within contexts, this Position Statement also emphasizes attending to social, physical, institutional, media and other contextual features that bound occupational choices and possibilities as people age.

The concept of occupational possibilities provides one way to analyse how contextual features come to bound what people can and cannot do based on particular social markers, such as age, disability or gender. Occupational possibilities refer to the 'ways and types of doing that come to be viewed as ideal and possible within a specific socio-historical context, and that come to be promoted and made available within environments' (Laliberte Rudman 2006, p.188). Over time, people in a specific social context come to view particular occupations as possible and ideal for themselves and for others on the basis of characteristics, such as specific diagnoses, and other occupations as not possible or inappropriate. These taken-for-granted assumptions about occupation are socially shaped through dominant discourses, broadly defined as ways of writing and talking about a particular group of people or social issue that circulate through everyday interactions, social policies, institutional policies, healthcare professional texts and guidelines, popular media and other systems and structures. Thus, these discourses not only shape how people understand what they and others should and should not do, but are also embedded in broader aspects of societies in ways that support and constrain occupations.

Whilst acknowledging that dementia can occur prior to 'old age', with some people diagnosed in their forties and fifties, we ask you to reflect on older adults, often defined as those aged 65 and above, as an example. Think about what is taken for granted about what older adults can and should do as they age. What occupations seem like the 'right' things for ageing adults to engage in, and towards what aims? What occupations are often portrayed as dangerous, inappropriate and immoral for ageing adults? Research analysing dominant ageing discourses in Western contexts have pointed to a strong distinction between ideals of 'positive' or 'successful ageing' and those of the 'fourth age' or 'advanced old age'. Dominant positive or successful ageing discourses, promoted by academics, policymakers and healthcare professionals, mark out an ideal construction of ageing characterized by the absence of disability, responsible lifestyle choices, continued independence and ongoing engagement in particular socially appropriate and health-promoting occupations (Laliberte Rudman 2006).

These ageing discourses have been welcomed, within and outside of occupational therapy, for potentially opening a greater range of occupational possibilities for later life. However, they have also been critiqued for a narrow focus on particular occupations, such as those tied to remaining youthful and staying productive, and for placing responsibility onto ageing individuals for managing the risks and challenges of their own ageing so as to maintain independence. Such discourses fail to consider inequitable access to the resources and conditions required to participate as a 'positive' ageing citizen, such as financial resources, adequate housing or absence of physical or cognitive impairments. Moreover, they create few occupational possibilities for ageing individuals who cannot live up to the ideals promoted – those who experience poverty, homelessness or disability, for example.

In combination with valorizing independence, concerns have been raised regarding how so-called 'positive' ageing discourses actually reproduce ageist assumptions, reinforcing taken-for-granted assumptions that becoming 'old', particularly in the sense of experiencing disability, necessarily leads to negative outcomes of dependency, incapability, medical management and loss of autonomy (Laliberte Rudman 2017; McParland, Kelly and Innes 2017; Trentham 2019). For example, a study of occupational therapists' discharge planning practices with older adults revealed that recommendations about appropriate discharge location were heavily influenced by discourses of ageing, with disability as a time of inevitable decline, in which physical safety should be prioritized over continued possibilities to engage in desired occupations in one's environment of choice (Njelesani *et al.* 2015). As another example, Trentham (2019) challenges the long-standing focus on independence in basic activities of daily living within occupational therapy practices with ageing people. Trentham raises concerns that a focus on independence may reinforce system-level needs to minimize the provision of care whilst neglecting ageing clients' occupational needs and desires.

When considering the everyday lives of people living with dementia, the concept of occupational possibilities provides a way for occupational therapists to question what has come to be taken for granted about what people with dementia should and should not do, within broader society, in healthcare and other systems, and by occupational therapists. Just as we can reflect on assumptions about age embedded in dominant discourses, we can also think about dominant discourses regarding people with dementia and their implications for occupational possibilities. For example, think about what assumptions you have about what occupations comprise the everyday lives of people with dementia, what occupations are risky for those with dementia, and moving to another level, what types of occupations tend to be prioritized and supported within contemporary healthcare systems for people with dementia, and what types of occupations might be neglected or restricted.

Whilst acknowledging the growth of discourses that emphasize possibilities for living well with dementia, biomedical discourses of dementia that construct it as a 'tragedy' continue to be dominant within some healthcare systems, popular media and academic discourse (Kontos 2005; McParland *et al.* 2017). Such tragedy discourses depict dementia as characterized by 'loss of function, decline and death' (McParland *et al.* 2017, p.258), constructing people with dementia as deviant, outside 'normal' society, incapable of practising citizenship, and as experiencing social death and loss of personhood (Bond, Corner and Graham 2004;

Kontos 2005; McParland *et al.* 2017). These tragedy discourses may limit the occupational possibilities of people with dementia in diverse ways. For example, they may face barriers to occupations due to social stigma perhaps experienced in the local community's attitudes and behaviours as well as exclusion from decision-making related to their occupations. As another example, within rehabilitation, tragedy discourses may lead to a deficit-focused approach, specifying how a person with dementia is impaired rather than highlighting their strengths and abilities to continue to enjoy diverse activities and social connection with others (Alzheimer's Disease International 2012). Moreover, O'Sullivan and Hocking (2013, p.174) acknowledge that there can be a tendency to identify only risks when working with people with dementia, but 'doing gives purpose to life and so the balance of risk must be carefully weighed to include the dignity of risk.'

Grounded in a rights-based perspective, there is a need for ongoing critical reflection on how taken-for-granted assumptions, circulated through discourses, may serve to exclude people with dementia from occupations that are meaningful and contribute to the wellbeing of themselves, their families and communities. In turn, it is important for occupational therapists to be part of efforts aimed at the social trans-formation of discourses, practice, systems and structures to support the occupational rights of people with dementia.

Social transformation through occupation

Given that the occupational possibilities of people with dementia are shaped through social forces, part of the role of occupational therapists, working in collaboration with people with dementia, their families and other important community stakeholders, involves enacting social transformation aimed at challenging taken-for-granted assumptions, embedded in discourses, practice, systems and structures, that result in occupational marginalization for people with dementia. Within occupational therapy, there is growing attention on enacting social transformation through occupation, based in recognition of the need to question how taken-for-granted aspects of contemporary societies produce and perpetuate occupational marginalization and inequities (Laliberte Rudman *et al.* 2019; van Bruggen 2020). Broadly defined, social transformation through occupation includes various approaches that use occupation to restructure discourses, practices, systems and structures so as to address occupational and social inequities.

Such approaches use occupation as a means for social transformation and also work with individuals and collectives to enhance possibilities for participatory citizenship and occupational engagement. Approaches to social transformation through occupation often involve working with a group, inclusive of people experiencing marginalization, and key stakeholders. Additionally, various levels and types of social change can be targeted, such as in discourses, practices, resource allocation and social relations, to enable a greater diversity of occupational possibilities (van Bruggen *et al.* 2020).

We now provide one example of an initiative that is seeking to challenge dominant discursive representations of dementia. This initiative engages those with dementia and counters taken-for-granted assumptions regarding occupational possibilities, opening up spaces to rethink and alternatively support the citizenship and occupational engagement of people with dementia.

Challenging dominant discourses and expanding occupational possibilities

The dignity of risk and the right to sustain occupations when living with dementia is captured in a published eBook by the Scottish Dementia Working Group (SDWG) (Alzheimer Scotland 2019; see Chapter 1, 'Occupation Matters to Me'). The eBook was developed as part of an Alzheimer Scotland occupational therapy internship project (see Chapter 10 in this book) developed in partnership with Queen Margaret University, Edinburgh. Informed by photovoice methodology, its purpose was to allow members of the SDWG the opportunity to adopt photography as a means through which they could represent the possibility and importance of sustaining occupations following a diagnosis of dementia.

The eBook was co-produced by those members of the SDWG who participated and the interns who were pre-, post- or recent graduates of occupational therapy at Queen Margaret University. The process of co-production included two key cornerstones of approach:

- First, recognition from the outset of the need to build on and visually represent the existing capabilities of participants. In so doing the photographs contributed to one outcome of the project, the creation of an eBook, to aid the ambition of the SDWG to act as agents of change.

• Second, the value and importance of reciprocity, which grew in strength as the project evolved. As the occupational therapy interns and the SDWG learned together and with each other, reciprocity was valued and appreciated, helping to create an environment of trust. For example, one member of the SDWG commented, 'When that photograph book came, it was really something special. I would never have thought about doing that.'

Similarly, an occupational therapy intern, reflecting on the process of partnership, noted, 'Working with the SDWG has enabled me to learn how to develop positive, well-supported partnerships. This is something I will take forward with me as a therapist.' In working to build together a trusting partnership, the photographs included in the eBook illuminate the value and importance of the 'everyday' way(s) we occupy our time, helping to maintain a sense of purpose and self-identity, including sustaining connection with communities, following a diagnosis of dementia.

The collection of photographs also represents a tool through which the centrality of occupation in the lives of people living with dementia has been harnessed to raise public awareness of the need to challenge a tendency towards a deficit-focused approach or taken-for-granted assumptions, restricting occupational possibilities. Instead, the photographs seek to give voice and expand the occupational possibilities of people living with dementia, and in so doing the eBook aims to influence change, including government-level dementia policy, how and in what way regional and organizational dementia services are constructed and delivered, and how families and people living with dementia can respond to their diagnosis.

This example illustrates how the ideas underpinning occupation-based social transformation can influence the design and implementation of initiatives that seek to promote the rights of people living with dementia, to sustain their occupational possibilities throughout all stages of the diagnosis (see also van Bruggen *et al.* 2020). Key ideas include:

- *Building partnerships:* We see the importance of the involvement of multiple partners across sectors and generations (in this case, a national third sector organization, a higher education institution, members of a representative group and students).
- *Reflexivity:* Doing the occupation (creation of an eBook) together offered a space for reflection and the creation of new knowledge for those taking part.
- *Flexibility and diversity:* The occupation itself supported the inclusion of people with a diverse range of knowledge and skills, acknowledging and celebrating their diversity.
- *Power:* Those people with the most knowledge of the issues, those with experience of living with dementia, were positioned at the heart of the initiative.

The outcome has the potential to reach and speak to diverse sectors (political, health and social care, educational), but also to homes and communities in Scotland and beyond. It challenges a traditional 'tragic' discourse by providing contrasting examples of the lived experiences of hope and possibility to sustain valued occupations when living with dementia.

Conclusion

Taking as a starting point the essentially social nature of our interconnected lives raises considerations for how we live together as citizens – how we 'do' and 'be' together. Age and dementia have been taken as examples of two intersecting axes of diversity that can shape what come to be seen as the 'right', ideal and healthy occupations for particular groups of people. These influence the occupational possibilities of these particular citizens, and are embedded in broader systems and structures, including occupational therapy practices, as well as their everyday lives in their communities.

Occupation can contribute to processes of social transformation, as through new or different opportunities for being and doing together we can not only create spaces for change for individuals and their community, but also challenge the taken-for-granted occupational possibilities of people with dementia.

Reflective questions

1. Identify collective occupations you engage in as a citizen (such as informal daily encounters, celebratory or commemorative occupations, organized/associations/advocacy occupations). In what ways do they contribute to the social world of which you are a part?

2. Over a few days, take a note of references to ageing and dementia that you observe in advertisements, television programmes, blog or twitter posts. What 'images' or 'messages' are being created about these groups of people (both positive and negative) and their occupational possibilities?

3. Reflecting on contemporary healthcare systems, what types of occupations tend to be prioritized and supported for people with dementia, and what types of occupations might be neglected or restricted?

4. Consider how a biomedical lens influences processes of referral assessment, treatment, etc. How might they change if influenced by an occupational lens?

References

Alzheimer's Disease International (2012) *World Alzheimer Report 2012: Overcoming the Stigma of Dementia*. London: Alzheimer's Disease International. Accessed on 22/04/2022 at www.alzint.org/resource/world-alzheimer-report-2012

Alzheimer Scotland (2019) *Occupation Matters to Me*. Edinburgh: Alzheimer Scotland. Accessed on 19/10/2021 at www.alzscot.org/sites/default/files/2019-12/SDWG%20 e-Book.pdf

Bartlett, R. and O'Connor, D. (2010) 'From personhood to citizenship: Broadening the lens for dementia practice and research.' *Journal of Aging Studies* 21, 107–118.

Bond, J., Corner, L. and Graham, R. (2004) 'Social Science Theory on Dementia Research: Normal Ageing, Cultural Representation and Social Exclusion.' In A. Innes, C. Archibald and C. Murphy (eds) *Dementia and Social Inclusion* (pp.220–236). London: Jessica Kingsley Publishers.

Hoskins, B., Abs, H., Han, C., Kerr, D. and Veugelers, W. (2012) *Contextual Analysis Report: Participatory Citizenship in the European Union*. Brussels: Institution of Education. Accessed on 19/10/2021 at http://ec.europa.eu/citizenship/pdf/ report_1_conextual_report.pdf

Kantartzis, S. and Molineux, M. (2017) 'Collective occupation in public spaces and the construction of the social fabric.' *Canadian Journal of Occupational Therapy 84*, 3, 168–177.

Kontos, P. (2005) 'Embodied selfhood in Alzheimer's disease: Rethinking person centred care.' *Dementia 4*, 4, 553–570.

Laliberte Rudman, D. (2006) 'Positive aging and its implications for occupational possibilities in later life.' *Canadian Journal of Occupational Therapy 73*, 3, 188–192.

Laliberte Rudman, D. (2017) 'The Duty to Age Well: Critical Reflections on Occupational Possibilities Shaped through Discursive and Policy Responses to Population Ageing.' In D. Sakellariou and N. Pollard (eds) *Occupational Therapies without Borders: Integrating Justice and Practice* (2nd edn, Chapter 35). London: Elsevier.

Laliberte Rudman, D., Pollard, N., Craig, C., Kantartzis, S., *et al.* (2019) 'Contributing to social transformation through occupation: Experiences from a think tank.' *Journal of Occupational Science 26*, 2, 316–322.

McParland, P., Kelly, F. and Innes, A. (2017) 'Dichotomising dementia: Is there another way?' *Sociology of Health & Illness 39*, 2, 258–269.

Njelesani, J., Teachman, G., Durocher, E., Hamdani, Y. and Phelan, S.K. (2015) 'Thinking critically about client-centred practice and occupational possibilities across the life-span.' *Scandinavian Journal of Occupational Therapy 22*, 4, 252–259.

O'Connor, D. and Nedlund, A.-C. (2016) 'Editorial introduction: Special Issue on Citizenship and Dementia.' *Dementia 15*, 3, 285–288.

O'Sullivan, G. and Hocking, C. (2013) 'Translating action research into practice: Seeking occupational justice for people with dementia.' *OTJR: Occupation, Participation and Health 33*, 3, 168–176.

Pollard, N., Kantartzis, S., Fransen-Jaïbi, H. and Viana-Moldes, I. (2021) 'Occupational Therapy on the Move: On Contextualizing Citizenships and Epistimicide.' In R.E. Lopes and A.P.S. Malfitano (eds) *Social Occupational Therapy: Theoretical Designs and Practical Outlines* (Chapter 15). Philadelphia, PA: Elsevier.

Trentham, B. (2019) 'Ageism and the valorization of independence: Are they connected?' *British Journal of Occupational Therapy 82*, 4, 199–200.

van Bruggen, H., Craig, C., Kantartzis, S., Laliberte Rudman, D., *et al.* (2020) *Case Studies for Social Transformation through Occupation*. European Network of Occupational Therapy in Higher Education. Accessed on 19/10/2021 at https://enothe. eu/wp-content/uploads/2020/06/ISTTON-booklet-final.pdf

WFOT (World Federation of Occupational Therapists) (2021) *Occupational Therapy and Ageing Across the Life Course*. Position Statement. London: WFOT. Accessed on 19/10/2021 at www.wfot.org/resources/ occupational-therapy-and-ageing-across-the-life-course

CHAPTER 7

Occupational Justice

Air Travel and People with Dementia

Alison Warren, Katherine Turner, Maria O'Reilly
and Ian Kenneth Grant Sherriff

Learning outcomes

By the end of this chapter, you will have the opportunity to:

- Explore air travel from an occupational perspective for people living with dementia and their caregivers
- Investigate the stages of the travel chain through strategic collaborative examples that highlight barriers and facilitators to air travel
- Gain an understanding of the legislation, policy and guidelines fundamental to empowering people living with dementia and their caregivers to travel by air
- Source practical strategies to enable air travel to support 'what people want, need and have the right to do' that is informed by stakeholder involvement, occupational therapists and research.

Introduction

It is estimated that by 2030, 82 million people will be living with dementia worldwide (Alzheimer's Disease International 2020), making the support of people living with dementia a global challenge. This indicates that the number of people travelling with cognitive changes, not all with a diagnosis of dementia, is likely to increase. It has been reported that air travel for people with dementia and their travel companions can at times prove challenging. There are particular points along what we describe in this text as the 'travel chain' that can present barriers, beginning with planning a trip, the journey from home, through airports, inflight and the return journey. Although there have been some improvements within infrastructure to meet the needs of travellers with physical disabilities, those living with dementia and other hidden disabilities had until more recently often gone unnoticed.

This chapter seeks to share research undertaken by occupational therapists in the UK and Australia in collaboration with key stakeholders to add to the growing evidence base to improve the flying experiences of people with dementia and their travel companions. Whilst this chapter focuses on the occupation of air travel for people living with dementia, the collaborative and strategic approach taken by occupational therapists with relevant stakeholders is transferrable to other occupational areas when working with service users.

So why is air travel of interest to occupational therapists?

Many of us engage in travel as an occupation in its own right as it enhances our wellbeing or as a means to access further meaningful occupations, for example, visiting friends, taking a holiday or completing work trips. Envisage a journey as a series of links in a chain – preparing and packing, getting to the airport, checking in...etc. Research shows us that this chain can be disrupted at any link; thus, the weakest link determines the outcome of the journey.

Imagine if you or someone you care about was prevented from taking a flight based purely on a diagnosis or because assistance may be required at different stages of the travel chain. At this point lack of access to this occupation would not feel right or just.

Occupational scientists introduced the concept of occupational justice as a means of promoting and enabling equitable participation in occupations (Durocher, Gibson and Rappolt 2014), although the sub-terms of occupational justice – deprivation, marginalization, alienation, imbalance and apartheid – have been criticized due to inconsistencies in their meaning and a lack of evidence to support their use across different cultures (Whalley Hammell and Beagan 2017). The World Federation of Occupational Therapists (WFOT) contend that occupational justice is essentially a person's right to choose, participate and engage in a range of meaningful occupations, with a breach of a person's occupational rights being a breach of their human rights (WFOT 2019). Mace *et al.* (2018) suggest that occupational justice is fundamentally a person's right and freedom to do what they want and need to do, and to be who they want and need to be.

Recognizing and upholding a person's human rights is central to occupational therapy research and practice. Indeed, it is suggested that as occupational therapists enable people to overcome barriers to participation, we are an inherently political profession (Pollard and Sakellariou 2014). Arguably, however, occupational therapists need to be much more proactive in highlighting and directly addressing occupational injustices by emphasizing a person's right to participate in activities that are meaningful to them (Whalley Hammell 2017). This is particularly important for people living with dementia, who may face infringement of their rights on a daily basis due to paternalistic attitudes and stigmatization surrounding what someone with dementia should look, sound and act like (Hare 2016). Political activism has been integral to our work on accessible aviation, as demonstrated in the two strategic collaborative examples within this chapter.

There are a growing number of research projects related to air travel for people with dementia that involve occupational therapists and occupational therapy students. This is not surprising given the interest in travel as an occupation and an awareness of how the travel chain may be challenging for many people, including those with a hidden disability. In addition, research focusing on the travel experience of people with dementia and airport and security staff in Australia (Edwards *et al.* 2016), shared later in this chapter, has been replicated in the UK context. These exploratory online surveys and qualitative interviews highlighted that people living with dementia do travel by air and experience challenges including wayfinding at the airport, accessing toilets and sensory overload from crowds and noise, and are not aware of any entitlement to assistance when travelling (O'Reilly and Shepherd 2016; Turner 2021). Further in-depth, qualitative research has informed the challenges and solutions outlined in this chapter. Our research has been informed by stakeholder involvement including people living with dementia, their caregivers, representatives from airports and airlines, aircrew trainers, security advisers, dementia charities, academics and health professionals, including occupational therapists.

Collaboration: sharing best practice and research

This section provides an overview of two collaborative projects and research involving occupational therapists and key stakeholders. Travelling by air is made up of various stages that, whilst enjoyable, can be complex and ever changing. With the increase in the use of automation, strict security requirements and the amount of time required to complete a journey, air travel can present challenges for all travellers, but in particular for those requiring assistance.

Through introducing key working groups, projects and research from Australia and the UK, challenges and solutions are highlighted here to successfully navigate the stages of the travel chain. Through collaboration, what started as local and regional projects have evolved into I-D-Air, an International Dementia Air Travel working group highlighting worldwide initiatives, sharing knowledge and best practice. People interested in joining this virtual group can contact us for further information.

Strategic collaborative example in the UK

It is well documented that political awareness can and will generate positive changes for individuals and their communities. It is said that behind every political headline lies a human story. In the case of the Prime Minister's Dementia Challenge Group for Air Transport in the UK, which formed in 2015, we were being told by people living with dementia and their families of the personal challenges and difficulties they faced when travelling by air in the UK. A family caregiver of a person living with dementia explained how they were separated going through security, which caused the relative to become disorientated and frightened, resulting in the holiday being cancelled. This situation was not because the security staff were overstepping their remit; it was because they were neither trained nor aware of how to support a person living with dementia in an airport setting at that time. This lack of awareness also applied to some other staff and retail outlets within the airport.

The chairperson of the Prime Minister's Dementia Challenge Group for Air Transport was given the remit to gain a better understanding of the challenges and solutions for people living with dementia and their families who wanted to travel by air, and to make it a pleasurable and safe experience. The Group included at different times people living with dementia and their families, airports and airline staff, pilots, tourism specialists, cabin crew, ground crew, security staff, academics from the

Universities of Plymouth and Bournemouth, and a PhD student who is an occupational therapist, whose thesis was on air travel for people living with dementia and their families. It was a truly diverse and knowledgeable cross-section of people.

The Group, with the support of the Minister of State for Transport, secured an adjournment debate in the House of Commons (UK Parliament 2016). This generated a lively and informed discussion by all sides of the House. The combined efforts of this debate and the many months of consultation, meetings, flying in a simulator, visiting airports and working collaboratively with the Civil Aviation Authority (CAA) has led to many positive outputs from the Group. Collaboration with the Group was key to the recent development of the CAA guidance for airports on providing assistance to people with hidden disabilities (CAP 1411, CAA 2016) and for airlines (CAP1603, CAA 2018). This meant that stakeholders, including people living with dementia, informed national guidance setting out how both airports and airlines must comply with obligations under Regulation EC1107/2006 concerning the rights of disabled people and people with reduced mobility (PRM). The term 'PRM' is often misleading, however, and can cause issues for people travelling with hidden disabilities including dementia, as highlighted by the cartoon shown later (see Figure 7.2). In one UK airport, there are plans to adopt the phrase and abbreviation 'people requiring support' (PRS), which will hopefully encourage more people to seek assistance and support when travelling. It will be interesting to see if this or similar phrases are adopted within the air industry and in legislation over the coming years. In addition, it is essential to seek further review and development of guidance by the CAA in the UK or equivalent organizations in other countries to keep this important topic on the international agenda.

Strategic collaborative example in Australia

In 2015, a group of researchers in Brisbane, Australia asked the question, 'Do people with dementia travel by plane, and what are their experiences when they do?' To answer that question, a series of online surveys for travellers with dementia, their travel companions and the staff they interacted with in airlines and airport security was developed. Follow-up interviews with some of the travel companions were also conducted. It was found that people with dementia were flying on average twice a year. The most common type of trip was international long-haul travel, and the most common reason to travel was for leisure. Most respondents reported they had experienced problems at the airport, such as finding restrooms and their boarding gate, hearing announcements, checking in, reading information on signboards and bag screening. Despite this, almost half of the travellers surveyed planned to continue travelling by air. Whilst challenges once on board their flights were reported, the surveys and interviews indicated that the most challenging part of the journey was at the airport, so the logical next step in our work was to investigate the physical and social environment of the airport to understand how it could better support travellers with dementia.

We were fortunate to develop a positive working relationship with Brisbane Airport Corporation, working closely with them to conduct a dementia-friendly audit of the domestic and international terminals, and through that process we were able to recommend changes that enabled the airport to become more dementia-inclusive. We used the Dementia Friendly Communities Environmental Assessment Tool (DFC-EAT) (Fleming and Bennett 2015). This allowed us to look closely at ways the airport space can facilitate or detract from a positive travel experience. Using the DFC-EAT allowed us to calculate a 'dementia-friendly' score for each segment of the travel chain through the airport. Like most airports across the globe, a private corporation runs Brisbane Airport, with the zones within the terminals controlled by different organizations. The complex commercial arrangements make it difficult to ensure consistency of design throughout the terminals. We recommended improvements to wayfinding signage and seating throughout the airport, colour and texture of flooring, quiet spaces and, importantly, enhancing the awareness of customer assistance.

The travel chain: challenges and solutions

Drawing from research, this section outlines a range of challenges experienced by people living with dementia and their companions when travelling by air, with suggestions for possible solutions. The air travel chain describes various points, beginning with planning a trip, the journey from home, through airports, inflight and the return journey. There are several stages involved that relate to landside, that is, before arriving and when in the airport, whilst airside relates to once through security and on the flight. There are many steps and tasks involved in this occupation, including booking a trip, arriving at the airport, car parking, navigating check-in, security and passport control as well as completing activities of daily living whilst confined in a small space for the flight.

Darcy (2012) highlighted that air travel practices routinely contravened disability discrimination legislation at various stages of the travel chain. This has been echoed in research and working group projects. More detailed air travel tips for people with dementia can be found in O'Reilly and Shepherd (2016) and Turner (2021). Here, we highlight some challenges experienced by people living with dementia and their families and describe potential solutions. The solutions will need to be addressed by a range of people including airports, airlines, those responsible for regulating air travel, legislators and health and social care professionals supporting those living with dementia. The greatest challenge is providing a cohesive response to ensure that all aspects are addressed, which ultimately has the potential to improve the air travel experiences of all passengers.

Pre-travel
Challenge: Knowing your rights to assistance and support before you travel.

Solution: Aviation regulators should enforce standards regarding assistance for people with dementia at airports and when travelling with airlines. Some changes have already been made in the UK and Australia to highlight that special assistance is available to passengers with hidden disabilities at airports, and hidden disability lanyards can be provided to indicate support might be required. Enhanced dementia awareness training is also required for landside and airside staff.

At the airport
Challenge: Separation of the travel companion and the person with dementia leading to difficulty comprehending complex instructions and sensory overload, such as going through security, using boarding cards and at passport control.

Solution: There must be greater acknowledgement of the role of the travel companion in supporting the person with dementia by facilitating people to travel together. For some, the use of a wheelchair may be helpful in reducing the cognitive load, with a member of staff to assist people through the airport checkpoints. Quiet routes and rooms in the airport can also reduce sensory overload in the airport environment. The use of colour should be considered, to make the environment accessible.

Adaptations can be made in the airport environment to make it easier to navigate. One example includes the use of colour in a glass lift in Brisbane International Airport. Figure 7.1 shows the glass lift, the design of which made it hard to find and identify. The simple addition of a yellow background behind the glass either side of the lift doors subsequently made the lift more visible.

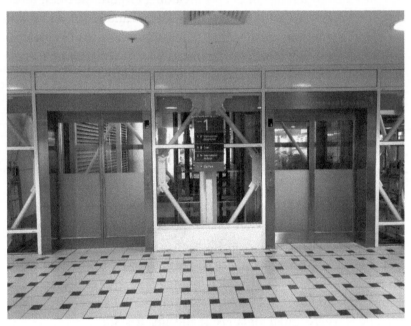

Figure 7.1. Glass lift at Brisbane International Airport

Boarding the aircraft
Challenge: Stepping on and off the aircraft and waiting in queues.

Solution: Give people the choice to board first or last so there is less pressure to find seats and stow hand luggage. Also, give people with visual-spatial difficulties time to move between changes in flooring at their own pace, and to receive any guidance required from their travel companion.

Inflight
Challenge: Using the toilets, which are generally in a confined space, with some unfamiliar equipment and door locks.

Solution: The passenger should seek advice from the aircrew team if they are concerned, so that the toilet can be accessed safely. Also, noise-cancelling headphones, comfortable clothing and a range of activities that can be completed when seated may be helpful, such as books, artwork and familiar music.

Arrival at destination
Challenge: Separating people when going through border control where language may also be an issue as well as the automation of some processes.

Solution: There must be greater acknowledgement of the role of the travel companion in supporting the person with dementia by facilitating people to travel together in all countries. Airport staff may need to be approached in the arrivals areas to gain support.

Return journey
Challenge: Checking in prior to departure for the journey home, as checking-in procedures may have changed and check-in kiosks can look different between airports.

Solutions: Ensure that the check-in procedures have been followed, as this may be required prior to arrival at the airport. Allow plenty of time to progress through the stages and seek assistance at automated checkpoints. Signage could be improved throughout airports to guide passengers through the different steps of the travel chain.

Strategic collaborative example: cartoons as discussion starters
Phenomenological interview findings as part of doctoral research by an occupational therapist highlighted the importance of air travel for some people living with dementia as well as key challenges (Turner 2021). Cartoons can be an accessible means of capturing and sharing the voices and experiences of people living with dementia (Beesley, Husband and McMillian 2018), and promote problem-solving through discussion.

Consequently, in 2020, a grant was awarded by the Plymouth Institute of Health and Care Research QR Strategic Priorities Fund to enable 12 of Tony Husband's cartoons to be commissioned based on the research findings.

Tony Husband is a UK-based, award-winning cartoonist who has utilized his artistic skills to depict his father's experiences of living with vascular dementia (Husband 2014). A stakeholder group for the doctoral research determined which of the research quotes should be turned into images, with each image portraying a specific challenge or challenges associated with a different section of the air travel chain. One of the final images from the series is shown in Figure 7.2. This research and the images informed the development of the pamphlet *Flying with Dementia: An Informative Guide*, containing top tips for air travel in collaboration with Heathrow airport (University of Plymouth and Heathrow 2021).

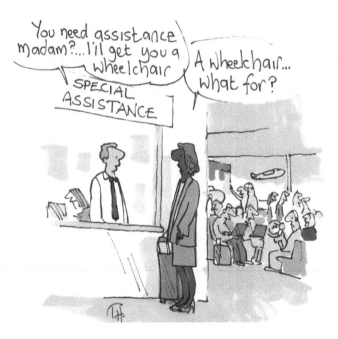

Figure 7.2. Challenges of special assistance for people with hidden disabilities
Source: Turner, Warren and Sherriff (2021), © University of Plymouth (2021)

Conclusion

Airports and airlines worldwide need to consider strategies for ensuring smooth journeys for travellers with dementia. As highlighted by Warren, Turner and Chami (2017), occupational therapists can take a lead role, working in partnership with stakeholders, to promote dementia-friendly travel initiatives to facilitate air travel as a meaningful occupation for people living with dementia. This chapter has also emphasized the value of working collaboratively at a local level to generate change nationally, and these principles can be applied to different occupational areas.

Making transport infrastructure accessible is an important part of increasing the self-determination and independence of people living with dementia. This chapter has shared research-informed practical strategies and ideas to enhance the travel chain experience. As occupational therapists and occupational therapy students using our core professional values of being person-centred, occupation-focused and advocates of occupational justice, we are invaluable members of active stakeholder groups. As a profession, we can use our holistic skills and creative problem-solving to assist with audits of the airport environment to promote accessible design as well as talking through practical solutions to facilitate individuals and their companions to continue travelling by air. Thinking more globally, the next steps involve encouraging membership of I-D-Air, to share successes, support the development of new dementia-friendly initiatives and facilitate the co-production of meaningful research.

By using a collaborative problem-solving approach between researchers, consumers and decision-makers, current and future projects also have the potential to continue to improve the travel experiences for all, and ensure the rights of passengers with both physical and hidden disabilities are upheld. As Kate Turner (2021, p.327) noted in her doctoral thesis:

> A simple way all occupational therapists could begin to engage in rights-based practice is to reframe their answer to the common question 'what is occupational therapy?', by stating that it is the practice of enabling a person to do the things they want, need, and have the right to do.

Reflective questions

1. What do you think is happening in the scenario depicted in Figure 7.2, and given what you have read in this chapter, do you think this passenger's rights are being upheld? Why or why not?
2. Consider the challenges and solutions highlighted earlier in the chapter. What will you do to uphold the rights of people to engage in travel as a meaningful occupation?
3. Thinking and acting locally, nationally and internationally, what steps will you take to facilitate people to travel by air?

Acknowledgements

The authors of this chapter would like to acknowledge the valuable contribution made by various working group members in Australia and the UK, research participants and occupational therapy students who undertook research related to air travel and people living with dementia. Research funding and support was provided through the Dementia Centre for Research Collaboration and Dementia Training Australia. We would like to acknowledge the contribution of those with lived experience who shared their expertise in reference groups and airport audits, and in particular, Christine and Paul Bryden, John Quinn and Glenys Petrie.

The School of Health Professions at the University of Plymouth funded the PhD studentship and the Plymouth Institute of Health and Care Research funded the innovative illustrations project to disseminate the findings to promote dementia-friendly flying. We would also like to acknowledge the Civil Aviation Authority, the Minister of State for Transport Oliver Colville MP, and members of the Prime Minister's Dementia Challenge Group for Air Transport, as without the hard work and sheer tenacity of these individuals and organizations, this work would not have made it off the drawing board.

References

Alzheimer's Disease International (2020) *Numbers of People with Dementia Around the World: An Update to the Estimates in the World Alzheimer Report 2015.* London:

Alzheimer's Disease International. Accessed on 01/12/2021 at www.alzint.org/resource/numbers-of-people-with-dementia-worldwide

Beesley, I., Husband, T. and McMillan, I. (2018) *The Right to a Grand Day Out*. Exeter: The Ideal Project. Accessed on 27/04/2022 at www.idealproject.org.uk/media/universityofexeter/schoolofpsychology/ideal/documents/A_Grand_Day_Out.pdf

CAA (Civil Aviation Authority) (2016) *Guidance for Airports on Providing Assistance to People with Hidden Disabilities*, CAP1411. Accessed on 01/12/2021 at https://publicapps.caa.co.uk/modalapplication.aspx?appid=11&mode=detail&id=7390

CAA (2018) *Guidance for Airlines on Assisting People with Hidden Disabilities*, CAP1603. Accessed on 01/12/2021 at www.caa.co.uk/News/Airlines-given-guidance-on-assisting-passengers-with-hidden-disabilities

Darcy, S. (2012) '(Dis) embodied air travel experiences: Disability, discrimination and the affect of a discontinuous air travel chain.' *Journal of Hospitality and Tourism Management 19*, 1–11, e8.

Durocher, E., Gibson, B.E. and Rappolt, S. (2014) 'Occupational justice: A conceptual review.' *Journal of Occupational Science 21*, 4, 418–430.

Edwards, H., O'Reilly, M., Beattie, E., Willmott, L. and Dreiling, A. (2016) *Infrequent Flyers? Exploring the Issue of Air Travel and Dementia from the Perspective of People with Dementia, their Carers, Airline Staff and Airport Services*. Queensland: Dementia Collaborative Research Centre.

Fleming, R. and Bennett, K.A. (2015) *Dementia Friendly Community Environmental Assessment Tool (DFC-EAT)*. Wollongong, NSW: University of Wollongong.

Hare, P. (2016) *Our Dementia, Our Rights*. Exeter: Innovations in Dementia CIC.

Husband, T. (2014) *Take Care, Son: The Story of my Dad and His Dementia*. London: Robinson.

Mace, J., Hocking, C., Waring, M., Townsend, L., *et al.* (2018) *Occupational Justice as the Freedom to Do and Be: A Conceptual Tool for Advocating for Human Rights*. Cape Town, South Africa: World Federation of Occupational Therapists Congress.

O'Reilly, M. and Shepherd, N. (2016) 'Making air travel easier for people with dementia.' *Australian Journal of Dementia Care 5*, 4, 24–25.

Pollard, N. and Sakellariou, D. (2014) 'The occupational therapist as a political being.' *Brazilian Journal of Occupational Therapy 22*, 3, 643–652.

Turner, K.A. (2021) 'Dementia Friendly Flying: Investigating the Accessibility of Air Travel for People Living with Dementia.' PhD Thesis, University of Plymouth [in submission].

Turner, K.A., Warren, A. and Sherriff, I. (2021) *Illustrations Project to Promote Dementia Friendly Flying*. Plymouth: Plymouth Institute of Health and Care Research, University of Plymouth.

UK Parliament (2016) *Hansard*, House of Commons Debates, 14 June 2016, vol. 611, col. 1729. Accessed on 01/12/2021 at https://hansard.parliament.uk/Commons/2016-06 14/debates/16061454000002/AirPassengersWithDementia?highlight=air%20travel#contribution-16061454000049

University of Plymouth and Heathrow (2021) *Flying with Dementia: An Informative Guide*. London: Heathrow. Accessed on 27/04/2022 at www.plymouth.ac.uk/uploads/production/document/path/21/21319/Heathrow_Dementia_Leaflet.pdf

Warren, A., Turner, K.A. and Chami, H. (2017) 'Working together to promote dementia friendly flying.' *OTnews*, February, 40–41.

WFOT (World Federation of Occupational Therapists) (2019) *Occupational Therapy and Human Rights (Revised)*. London: WFOT. Accessed on 22/04/2022 at www.wfot.org/resources/occupational-therapy-and-human-rights

Whalley Hammell, K.R. (2017) 'Opportunities for well-being: The right to occupational engagement.' *Canadian Journal of Occupational Therapy 84*, 4–5, 209–222.

Whalley Hammell, K.R. and Beagan, B. (2017) 'Occupational injustice: A critique.' *Canadian Journal of Occupational Therapy 84*, 1, 58–68.

CHAPTER 8

Digital Health Technology and Occupational Engagement

Fiona Fraser, Toni M. Page, Hannah Bradwell,
Katie Edwards and Alison Warren

Learning outcomes

By the end of this chapter, you will have the opportunity to:

▸ Explore the context and drivers of current occupational therapy practice and the need to engage with the digital health agenda

▸ Identify examples of how digital health technology can be used to enhance the lives of people living with dementia and their caregivers

▸ Reflect on some of the ethical, moral and professional dilemmas that may need to be considered when utilizing technology.

Context

Occupational therapy is a profession that advocates for the use of person-centred problem-solving and innovation in practice. Over recent decades, this creativity has moved towards the integration of technological solutions to facilitate engagement in occupations and support people to participate in their communities. At times advances in technology have been met with scepticism. For example, replacing home visits with virtual visits may be perceived as a threat by occupational therapists (Read *et al.* 2020), as advocating for the wellbeing, privacy and rights of individuals on virtual platforms may be viewed as challenging, whereas others within the profession have championed the use of technology to support all aspects of the occupational therapy process, and in particular, to support people living with dementia and their caregivers. This chapter seeks to encourage occupational therapists to consider ways in which digital technology can be introduced into professional practice.

Technological advances and solutions are ever changing, and so this chapter is not seeking to cover all areas. The focus is to share examples of how digital health technology can be used to enhance the lives of people living with dementia and their caregivers. It is also intended to encourage reflection on some of the dilemmas that may need to be considered as part of professional reasoning when utilizing technology.

Digital technologies are electronic systems, devices, tools and resources that generate, store or process data (Table 8.1 provides some examples of these). Digital technologies are used every day and have become inseparable from health and social care. The term 'digital health' has been described as an umbrella term encompassing a wide range of technologies, including eHealth, mHealth, telehealth, telecare, virtual reality, genomics, artificial intelligence (AI) and more (WHO 2019).

The Topol Review refers to the healthcare workforce needing to develop the skills and attitudes to empower service users in using digital health technologies to enhance their health and wellbeing (Topol 2019). Technologies can support people in taking more responsibility for their healthcare, and ensure they have the knowledge and skills to manage their health conditions (Coulter and Collins 2011; NHS 2019), and also offer support to those in caregiver roles.

Table 8.1. Example technologies from the Topol Review (2019)

Telemedicine/telecare
Smartphone apps
Sensors and wearables for diagnostics and remote monitoring
Virtual and augmented reality
Automated image interpretation using artificial intelligence (AI)
Interventional and rehabilitative robotics – socially assistive robots
Predictive analytics using artificial intelligence (AI)

As highlighted by the World Federation of Occupational Therapists (WFOT) and others (2017), as technology evolves there is a need for occupational therapists to become involved in the development and implementation of assistive devices with a technology focus to facilitate engagement in occupation. The profession has invaluable core skills, including occupational analysis and working collaboratively to seek creative solutions. This is evident with occupational therapists and students becoming involved with the Centre for Health Technology at the University of Plymouth and the Lab4Living at Sheffield Hallam University, two examples that we are familiar with. Occupational therapists and occupational therapy students can make a valuable contribution to promoting healthy ageing and participation in everyday life.

The Alzheimer's Society (2020) undertook a survey (n=2000) across the UK of people living with or impacted by dementia. The finding indicated that isolation caused by the COVID-19 pandemic demonstrated a reduction in conversations between people and an increased sense of loneliness. This reinforces the need to embrace person-centred technological solutions to reach out to those who may feel isolated as well as promoting independence and wellbeing. It is important for the profession of occupational therapy to embrace technological advances whilst still critiquing its use to maximize individual engagement in occupation.

Technology in the home

The need to engage with technology in its various forms is now very much part of everyday life. Whilst some technology can present challenges to individuals experiencing a decline in their cognitive functioning, there is evidence that some technology within the home environment can maintain occupational engagement and participation. Assistive technology devices and systems are well established, such as clocks, calendars, automatic lights, extreme temperature sensors, flood detectors and fall sensors that send notifications to mobile devices to indicate when movement has been detected. In addition, automatic pill dispensers enable someone to have a sense of independence whilst also managing potential risk.

More recently, the introduction of smart technology onto the market has added to the range of products that, whilst not designed specifically to address some of the challenges associated with dementia, have the potential to promote independence. Smartphones, tablets, remote heating controls, smoke and carbon dioxide detectors, smart watches and even household appliances such as smart washing machines and fridges are now commonplace. A smart washing machine will detect the fabric type and level of cleaning required, and set the programme accordingly. There are watches available that have integrated fall detection monitoring. A smart fridge can offer the user a 'live' camera image of the items in their fridge via the associated smartphone application, enabling someone to check what they have in their fridge whilst out doing their shop. Smart speakers also have the potential to act as a virtual diary, providing audio reminders as well as taking on the role of voice-enabled virtual assistants, answering questions or confirming the date or time. In addition, smart speakers have the potential to provide forms of entertainment, such as playing music or audiobooks or running through a quiz (Edwards *et al.* 2021).

Our ability to maintain social relationships and connections (see Chapter 5) has the potential to influence our health and wellbeing. It could be argued that for individuals experiencing a decline in their cognitive functioning, this need is even greater. Conversations and interactions with both familiar and new people all provide a unique form of cognitive stimulation. However, the impact of dementia can make the maintenance of these relationships more challenging. This may be due to logistical issues such as having to stop driving or a loss of confidence. This has promoted research into the potential role that social media can play in supporting individuals to maintain social connections they may have otherwise lost (Cornejo, Tentori and Favela 2013). The sharing of pictures and videos is a simple way to keep family and friends connected with visual cues, such as the names of people, clearly displayed, adding subtle but effective prompts.

As a consequence of the COVID-19 pandemic, the use of in-home technology has meant an expansion of telehealth. For people living with dementia, this has seen the development of cognitive stimulation therapy (CST) delivered through a range of online platforms, which means individuals no longer need to attend a physical venue, and CST can be delivered in a meaningful, familiar location. Whilst CST is not a new intervention, this new method of delivery has opened alternative ways to engage people who previously may not have felt as comfortable participating in a face-to-face environment, and could be expanded to encompass occupation-focused interventions. However, whilst this can be seen as a development, online therapy brings both challenges and opportunities. Careful planning and facilitation is vital not only to use time online effectively, but also to ensure the safety of online participants.

Technology promoting community participation

Continuing to participate in life beyond the home can be an essential element to someone's quality of life. Whether this is a gentle walk or a trip to the local shops, maintaining engagement and participation in activities outside the home can provide meaningful routine and purpose. Technology can play a role in promoting opportunities for community engagement.

The integration of location tracking into smartphones and watches can now support the navigation around someone's local community through tools such as maps and landmark identification. A range of stand-alone Global Positioning Systems (GPS)-enabled devices are available on the market that have the potential to maintain independence and confidence, and provide additional reassurance to people living with dementia and their caregivers. The devices can serve different purposes depending on the individual – for example, as a reminder to provide reassurance if a person feels unsure of their surroundings – or they can help to locate someone or provide a predetermined travel zone that sends an alert if the person travels beyond the set parameters.

Whilst these devices can facilitate community participation, there are naturally limitations. One of the obvious limitations of any wearable technology is the reality that they can be easily removed or left at home. Equally, if an item is hard to use or unappealing, engagement can be limited. Gathercole *et al.* (2021) highlighted that people living with dementia may need their caregivers to adapt and incorporate assistive technology into their everyday activities. This qualitative study exploring how people engage with assistive technology and telecare went on to acknowledge that technology might not necessarily enable someone to independently live at home for longer or mitigate against carer burden or anxiety. It acknowledged that many factors are involved that facilitate remaining at home that are beyond the remit of technology. Therefore, it is important to establish realistic goals in terms of the implementation of assistive technology to manage the expectations of everyone involved.

Technology in care homes

Occupational therapy can provide important interventions for people living with dementia in care homes, and some of these interventions may take the form of health technologies. The list of potential technology is endless and ever changing, so within this section we focus on some key research or projects. With people living with dementia being supported in a range of care facilities, from supported housing to residential and nursing homes, there is a growing need to provide interventions that are meaningful, promote wellbeing and are not staff resource-intensive.

Technologies that are becoming popular in care environments that deserve a review by occupational therapists are the use of smart speakers (Box 8.1), digital health kiosks (Box 8.2) and socially assistive robots (Box 8.3), as well as technology that promotes social interaction through sensory stimulation and games such as interactive surfaces. These examples add to the current range of assistive devices related to managing risk – for example pressure mats that trigger an alarm when someone steps on the mat – and require ongoing review.

Socially assistive robots (SARs) are a subfield of robotics including social, service and rehabilitation robots that assist individuals through social interaction (Feil-Seifer and Matarić 2005). Social robots hold huge potential in working alongside practitioners in meeting the increasing demand in care environments. Tobis *et al.* (2017) surveyed occupational therapy students (n=26) on their perceptions towards robots in the care of community-dwelling older people. They perceived robots as a useful assistant, particularly in providing emergency alarms, health parameter monitoring, cognitive training, exercise and medication or hydration reminders (Tobis *et al.* 2017). Humanoid robots (robots shaped like people) receive much research interest for their potential in care and rehabilitation as they can interact with individuals and groups, for example to facilitate exercise. Beyond the subtype of purely social robots, there is a range of physically assistive robots that may hold future potential in promoting independence, for example a robotic arm on ceiling rails to assist someone who is restricted in their movement.

Box 8.1. Smart speakers for increasing participation amongst care home residents with cognitive decline (dementia)

Much research in the area of technology-enabled care focuses on cutting-edge technologies that are still under development (Edwards *et al.* 2021), but some already commercially available products may improve the quality of life of those living with dementia. One example is smart speakers, devices that are voice-activated and often include a digital assistant that can perform interactive actions.

In one project, smart speakers were given to 150 residential care homes across Cornwall and the Isles of Scilly (Edwards *et al.* 2021). The aim was to understand if using smart speakers within care homes, including for people with dementia, could be 'normalized' or become a routine part of everyday life.

Some of the key benefits of having a smart speaker in the care home were enhanced engagement amongst residents with home activities, enjoyment, calming effects and the acquisition of new skills. These are important findings, as they show that affordable devices, such as smart speakers, that are readily available to buy, can be of benefit to care home residents, including those with dementia.

Here is an example of feedback from one care home about how the introduction of the smart speaker helped one of their residents: 'For me personally the most surprising and emotional moment was when one of our non-verbal residents chose Elvis Presley songs and sang together with Alexa. She had to sit in front of the Echo Spot to read lyrics of some of the songs, but she actually sang' (quoted in Edwards *et al.* 2021).

Box 8.2. Digital health kiosks

Digital health kiosks are devices that provide access to services including health information, clinical measurement collection (such as blood pressure), patient self-check-in, telemonitoring and teleconsultation. They have become an increasingly important part of everyday life. For example, think about the last time you went to an airport or a bank – quite often you need to use a kiosk to check in for a flight or to bank a cheque. Hospitals and GP surgeries are also now starting to use kiosks to provide information and check-ins for appointments. Kiosks for telehealth have been implemented in residential homes for older adults and include measures of cognitive performance and the opportunity for residents to engage with educational videos and 'brain fitness' games. Health information collected by the kiosks can be transmitted electronically to relevant healthcare professionals who can monitor ongoing conditions such as hypertension (Resnick *et al.* 2012) and cognitive decline (Thompson *et al.* 2011). This evidence suggests that kiosk use amongst older adults could provide meaningful activity, health improvement and the ability to monitor disease progression.

Box 8.3. Socially assistive robots (pets)

Animal-assisted therapy is generally thought to be beneficial for improving physical and psychological wellbeing, although some contexts make interventions with live animals challenging. For example, animals pose a risk of bites, scratches, allergies and infections, limiting their safety for older people living in residential care (Hung *et al.* 2019). For people with dementia, associated behavioural and psychological symptoms may also pose a risk to the animal (Soler *et al.* 2015). As a safe alternative, robot pets were developed as a psychosocial tool to support wellbeing for older adults and people with dementia.

The most well-researched companion robot is a robot harp seal, generally supported to produce therapeutic benefits (Hung *et al.* 2019). The literature suggests benefits in enhancing wellbeing, including reduced agitation, depression, stress, loneliness and reduced care provider burden (Hung *et al.* 2019). Interaction with the robot seal has also been shown to decrease psychotropic and analgesic medication use (Hung *et al.* 2019). This outcome is particularly relevant due to the detrimental impact of pharmacological treatments for older adults, including negative side effects and an increased risk of cardiac events and mortality.

A challenge with the robot seal, however, is the cost, which can limit its use in real-world practice. However, more affordable animatronic pets, such as interactive cats and dogs, may hold potential for use in future practice for older people. Previous work suggested these affordable devices may be even better received by older adults (Bradwell *et al.* 2019), to further promote similar wellbeing outcomes such as improvements in mood and affect, communication, social interaction and companionship (Koh *et al.* 2021). Such devices provide an engaging meaningful activity. The importance of meaningful activity cannot be over-stated for older people and for those with dementia, improving their physical and mental wellbeing (Smith *et al.* 2018).

Practical and professional considerations

To balance the obvious opportunities technology offers people living with dementia and their caregivers, it is important to also acknowledge the ethical, moral and professional dilemmas that can emerge when using technology in practice. Despite the encouraging results suggesting robots could provide practitioners with technological tools to improve wellbeing, engagement, independence and health for older people and people with dementia, their use is not without challenges and should be considered.

Commonly discussed concerns include affordability, infantilization (treating older people like children), deception (robots can be perceived as real by those with dementia), reduced human contact, intrusions on privacy and the use of collated data. As there appears to be a lack of consensus on the ethics of robots for older people at present, the following factors are worth consideration by practitioners:

- Are robot pets and companions infantilizing for older people?
- Are robots (that look like people or animals) deceiving older people with dementia?
- Would the use of robots to care for people, deliver therapies and exercise classes and promote independence reduce human contact? To what extent is this problematic?

It is likely that practitioners will need to conduct their own risk assessment and corresponding health and safety checks, including infection control strategies, when using technology and robotics to support their practice, particularly when considering any technology intended for shared use. In addition, there are also significant data sharing and privacy concerns associated with voice-activated devices, such as smart speakers (Lau *et al.* 2018). For example, when implemented into care homes some returned the smart speakers to research teams over concerns regarding access to confidential information (Edwards *et al.* 2021).

Apps and devices that provide feedback on an individual's location potentially highlight some further ethical dilemmas. Consideration needs to be given as to whether someone has the capacity to make an informed decision and can consent to wear technology that may provide helpful data on their whereabouts whilst simultaneously compromising their basic human right to privacy and sense of autonomy. It is necessary to weigh up the ethical principles of autonomy and having respect for an individual's freedom and privacy against beneficence (to do good) and non-maleficence (to do no harm). The right choice for those involved will be about striking a balance between potential intrusion and loss of dignity, an individual's right to take risks, and the benefits in terms of safety. Alongside these challenges, it should also be acknowledged that whilst technology provides many opportunities, we should strive to ensure the application of technology is not to the detriment of the personal and emotional contact an individual might need. Equally, the assumption should not be made that everyone has equal access to the technology described.

Conclusion

Although the future is unknown, one thing is clear – with the rate at which technology is developing, we are confident that more opportunities will become available that have the potential to support people living with dementia and their caregivers. There are opportunities for occupational therapists to engage in a wide range of research investigating the use of technology for people living with dementia, such as the INDUCT programme (Interdisciplinary Network for Dementia Using Current Technology). This aims to develop a multidisciplinary, intersectorial educational research framework across Europe to produce evidence demonstrating how technology can improve the lives of people with dementia. These educational providers have formed a Centre for Health Technology and are delivering projects to champion the development of a range of health innovations. The onus, however, will be on occupational therapists to remain aware of these developments and to identify the most appropriate application for these technologies. Whether it be utilizing different forms of extended reality or following the development of driverless cars, remaining cognisant of both the opportunities and challenges presented by technology has the potential to be an important strand to any continuing professional development activities.

Reflective questions

1. What technologies have you used or observed being used within health, social and community care settings, and could these be used to support people living with dementia?
2. How might the examples of health technologies that you can think of be used to support a person living with dementia or their caregiver's engagement in meaningful occupation?
3. What do you think are some of the key benefits and challenges when introducing technologies such as smart speakers to people living with dementia?
4. What further technologies could be developed that are aimed at supporting people living with dementia that promote wellbeing and participation?

References

Alzheimer's Society (2020) *The Impact of COVID-19 on People Affected by Dementia.* London: Alzheimer's Society. Accessed on 22/04/2022 at www.alzheimers.org.uk/sites/default/files/2020-08/The_Impact_of_COVID-19_on_People_Affected_By_Dementia.pdf

Bradwell, H.L., Edwards, K.J., Winnington, R., Thill, S. and Jones, R.B. (2019) 'Companion robots for older people: Importance of user-centred design demonstrated through observations and focus groups comparing preferences of older people and roboticists in South West England.' *British Medical Journal Open 2019,* 9, e032468. doi:10.1136/bmjopen-2019-032468

Cornejo, R., Tentori, M. and Favela, J. (2013) 'Enriching in-person encounters through social media: A study on family connectedness for the elderly.' *International Journal of Human-Computer Studies 71*, 9, 889–899.

Coulter, A. and Collins, A. (2011) *Making Shared Decision-Making a Reality: No Decision about Me without Me*. London: The King's Fund. Accessed on 01/03/2017 at www. kingsfund.org.uk/sites/default/files/Making-shared-decision-making-a-reality-paper-Angela-Coulter-Alf-Collins-July-2011_0.pdf

Edwards, K.J., Jones, R.B., Shenton, D., Page, T., *et al.* (2021) 'The use of smart speakers in care home residents: Implementation study.' *Journal of Medical Internet Research 23*, 12, e26767, doi:10.2196/26767.

Feil-Seifer, D. and Matarić, M. (2005) *Defining Socially Assistive Robotics. Proceedings of the 2005 IEEE International Conference on Rehabilitation Robotics*. Chicago, IL, 465–468. doi:10.1109/ICORR.2005.1501143

Gathercole, R., Bradley, R., Harper, E., Davies, L., *et al.* (2021) 'Assistive technology and telecare to maintain independent living at home for people with dementia: The ATTILA RCT.' *Health Technology Assessment 25*, 19.

Hung, L., Liu, C., Woldum, E., Au-Yeung, A., *et al.* (2019) 'The benefits of and barriers to using a social robot PARO in care settings: A scoping review'. *BMC Geriatrics 19*, 1, 232. doi:10.1186/s12877-019-1244-6

Koh, W.Q., Ang, F.X.H. and Casey, D. (2021) 'Impacts of low-cost robotic pets for older adults and people with dementia: Scoping review.' *JMIR Rehabilitation Assistive Technology 12*, 8, 1, e25340. doi:10.2196/25340

Lau, J., Zimmerman, B. and Schaub, F. (2018) 'Alexa, are you listening? Privacy perceptions and concerns and privacy-seeking behaviors with smart speakers.' *Proceedings of the Association of Computing Machinery on Human-Computer Interaction 2*, 102, 31. https://doi.org/10.1145/3274371

NHS (National Health Service) (2019) *The NHS Long Term Plan*. Accessed on 09/02/2019 at www.longtermplan.nhs.uk/wp-content/uploads/2019/08/nhs-long-term-plan-version-1.2.pdf

Read, J., Jones, N., Fegan, C., Cudd, P., *et al.* (2020) 'Remote home visit: Exploring the feasibility, acceptability and potential benefits of using digital technology to undertake occupational therapy home assessments.' *British Journal of Occupational Therapy 83*, 10, 648–658. doi:10.1177/0308022620921111

Resnick, H.E., Ilagan, P.R., Kaylor, M.B., Mehling, D. and Alwan, M. (2012) 'TEAhM – Technologies for Enhancing Access to Health Management: A pilot study of community-based telehealth.' *Telemedicine and e-Health 18*, 3, 166–174. doi:10.1089/tmj.2011.0122

Smith, N., Towers, A., Palmer, S., Beecham, J. and Welch, E. (2018) 'Being occupied: Supporting "meaningful activity" in care homes for older people in England.' *Ageing & Society 38*, 11, 2218–2240. doi:10.1017/S0144686X17000678

Soler, M.V., Aguera-Ortiz, L., Rodriguez, J.O., Rebolledo, C.M., *et al.* (2015) 'Social robots in advanced dementia.' *Frontiers in Ageing Neuroscience 7*, 133. doi:10.3389/fnagi.2015.00133

Thompson, H.J., Demiris, G., Rue, T., Shatil, E., *et al.* (2011) 'A holistic approach to assess older adults' wellness using e-health technologies.' *Telemedicine and e-Health 17*, 10, 794–800. doi:10.1089/tmj.2011.0059

Tobis, S., Cylkowska-Nowak, M., Wieczorowska-Tobis, K., Pawlaczyk, M. and Suwalska, A. (2017) 'Occupational therapy students' perceptions of the role of robots in the care of older people living in the community.' *Occupational Therapy International*, 1–6. doi.org/10.1155/2017/9592405

Topol, E. (2019) *The Topol Review: Preparing the Healthcare Workforce to Deliver the Digital Future*. Accessed on 08/09/2021 at https://topol.hee.nhs.uk

WFOT (World Federation of Occupational Therapists), Mackenzie, L., Coppola, S., Alvarez, L., *et al.* (2017) 'International occupational therapy research priorities.' *OTJR: Occupation, Participation and Health 37*, 2, 72–81.

WHO (World Health Organization) (2019) *Recommendations on Digital Interventions for Health System Strengthening – Research Considerations*. WHO Guideline. Geneva: WHO. Accessed on 22/04/2022 at www.who.int/publications/i/item/WHO-RHR-19.9

CHAPTER 9

Occupational Opportunities for People Living with Advanced Dementia

Angela Gregory and Margaret Brown

Learning outcomes
By the end of this chapter, you will have the opportunity to:

▸ Develop a deeper understanding of the possible occupational needs of a person living with advanced dementia

▸ Explore the evidence for a range of occupations to engage the person with advanced dementia, enhancing their health and wellbeing

▸ Acknowledge different perspectives when using occupational assessments and measuring outcomes

▸ Examine how everyday sensory, creative and embodied (that is, connected with the physical body) experiences could contribute to meaningful activity for the person with advanced dementia.

Introduction

This chapter intends to give the reader an overview of the possible occupational needs of people living with advanced dementia and to introduce the current considerations for practice. The content of the chapter and the practical activities suggested aim to inspire a creative approach to working with people with advanced dementia, support new learning and ultimately improve practice. We intend to highlight the importance of generating opportunities for meaningful engagement on behalf of the person with advanced dementia to ultimately celebrate their strengths and enhance their quality of life and everyday experiences.

We define the spectrum of dementia through an occupational lens, exploring how living with advanced dementia may affect a person's day-to-day living, wellbeing, relationships, roles and routines within their environment. Exploring occupational assessments, interventions and measuring outcomes sets the scene for discussing how people with advanced dementia may benefit from a sensory, creative and embodied approach.

What is advanced dementia?

There are over 100 different types of dementia that affect individuals in different ways depending on their life experiences, interests, preferred occupations and surrounding networks within their social and physical environment. Despite this diversity, dementia can often be described using a series of stages, ranging from mild or moderate to advanced. Although these stages contradict a person-centred ethos, they can provide a general sense of how occupations may need to be adapted, and may be useful when communicating with others who understand these terms. Occupational therapists can adapt this biomedical approach by using alternative perspectives such as the 'reflective, symbolic, sensorimotor and reflex' model (Perrin, May and Anderson 2008) and the 'planned, exploratory, sensory and reflex' levels (Pool 2012).

In this chapter, the term 'people living with advanced dementia' is used to describe a group of people living in the later stages of dementia (in some cases, for up to ten years) who are not yet near the end of life (Holmerova *et al.* 2016). This long period can be misperceived as unproductive, with people seemingly unresponsive, resulting in opportunities being reduced or missed, affecting their quality of life and wellbeing (Holmerova *et al.* 2016).

An occupational perspective of advanced dementia

People with advanced dementia have complex needs, which may go unnoticed and unmet. All aspects of a person's daily life will change, and the person will eventually require assistance with washing and dressing, eating and drinking, mobilizing and going to the toilet (Jack-Waugh *et al.* 2020). In their seminal work, Perrin, May and Anderson (2008) discuss how these difficulties are often due to deterioration in executive functioning, memory, language, movement and sensory processing. Therefore, occupational approaches would benefit from a bio-psycho-social-spiritual framework (Holmerova *et al.* 2016).

A person with advanced dementia may have a range of unmet needs, for example positioning to enable social and occupational engagement, and to facilitate safe eating and drinking. It is important to have an integrated person-centred and relational approach that encapsulates specialist knowledge and skills. Occupational therapists, and the person with advanced dementia and their family members, collaborate with a range of care professionals. These include care or nursing assistants, physiotherapists, speech and language therapists, psychologists, dieticians, podiatrists, nurses and doctors. This integrated approach to the person's needs is crucial in the advanced stages to optimize and maintain their remaining strengths for as long as possible.

As an activity we recommend watching a video from the Social Care Institute for Excellence (SCIE) (2014) featuring people living with advancing dementia and their families. Perhaps pay particular attention to Judy and her daughter to consider their occupational needs. To assist you, think of an occupational therapy model and adapt it in a format you have not tried before – you could use objects, drawings, mind maps, photographs or a collage to represent and explore occupations that may be of interest to Judy, Judy and her daughter, and Judy and staff within the care home setting. In practice, models are often service-led, but we would like you to think about which model suits Judy and her personal circumstances. We also recommend identifying the limitations of your chosen model to obtain an understanding of its usefulness.

A person living with advanced dementia can be underestimated in terms of their awareness and preserved skills. A thorough occupational, person- and relationship-centred assessment is required to establish environmental enablers and barriers, collate the person's life history, and understand their current interests, strengths, needs and challenges. Once these are known, the environment and occupation can be adapted to promote the person's current curiosities and abilities, empowering them to do some aspects of an occupation themselves, or be part of it. We have noticed that instinctive, protective actions by others can undermine the person's remaining abilities and selfhood. Therefore, it is important for occupational therapists to advocate for the person and to communicate effectively to others, demonstrating ways to maximize the involvement of the person living with advanced dementia to enhance their autonomy and maintain their personhood (see also Chapter 4).

Depending on the type of dementia and the individual, a person may also experience changes in their emotional state, personality and/or behaviour (Perrin *et al.* 2008) – for example, they may become anxious and appear agitated. Whilst repetitive behaviour may be interpreted as agitation, it is important not to make assumptions and to explore this further before any interventions are implemented, as this may essentially be a soothing occupation (Souyave *et al.* 2019). Folding occupations such as folding paper, clothes and everyday items are potentially meaningful, comforting and calming for people living with advanced dementia (Souyave *et al.* 2019). Premature decisions about the purpose of the person's actions may result in them being denied a meaningful opportunity. An occupational perspective is required to support the person to do the things that interest them at that time. It is therefore important to consider the meaning and purpose of the occupation and the person's innate and unique skills when facilitating opportunities (Wilcock and Hocking 2015), and not to 'prescribe' activities rigidly, as one size does not fit all.

Positive non-verbal communication is vital to use the person's strengths (Jack-Waugh *et al.* 2020). Adaptive interaction (Ellis and Astell 2017) and music-informed exchanges (Wood 2019) are alternative approaches to communication. Adaptive interaction imitates the gestures, vocalizations and facial expressions of people living with advanced dementia, aiming to provide acknowledgement and validation (Ellis and Astell 2017). Wood (2019) used a musical methodology to listen to conversations between people living with advanced dementia and their carer during self-care occupations like mealtimes. He analysed the pitch, tone and rhythm of their voices, finding importance in listening to the emotion and personality in the person's voice rather than the content, to create meaningful connections. A similar activity for you might be listening to a podcast or watching your favourite programme, for example, and instead of listening to the words, focus on the tones, rhythm and emotions of each person's voice. Reflect on what you 'hear' without words – do you recognize the emotions, feelings and expressions of the people involved?

Studies highlight that around 70 per cent of a person with advanced dementia's waking time is spent unoccupied in a care home (see Ellis and Astell 2017). Most interactions in a care home happen during personal care tasks, resulting in occupational and social needs being overlooked (Ellis and Astell 2017). This potentially breaches occupational justice, and is a situation that needs improvement and change. 'Occupational injustice' is a debateable term, described by Whalley Hammell and Beagan (2017) as having unequal access to occupations – a situation that can result in boredom, distress and dissatisfaction for a person living with advanced dementia (Brown *et al.* 2020). An alternative strengths-based, human rights approach (Whalley Hammell and Beagan 2017) can encourage practitioners to provide opportunities for creative, sensory-based and per-sonalized occupation (Brown *et al.* 2020). Occupational therapists are well placed to collaborate with and support care staff to increase their skills in enhancing occupational performance and to learn from one another.

Assessments and measuring outcomes

Standardized assessments can be used to determine the occupational performance of people with advanced dementia, for example the Pool Activity Level (PAL) Instrument for Occupational Profiling (Pool 2012) (see also Chapter 13) and the Model of Human Occupation Exploratory Level Outcome Ratings (MOHO-ExpLOR) (Cooper *et al.* 2018). We encourage you to familiarize yourself with different assessments to explore their strengths and limitations for this group of people – perhaps try them with a peer to build your confidence in using them.

The optimum approach to gathering information for assessment is being or doing with the person, sensitively observing the person, talking to the person's family members or friends, and discussing the person's strengths and needs with the wider team. Although it is important to understand the person's past interests and life history, it is essential to find out the person's current preferences as they may respond spon-taneously, in the moment. Assessing a person over a period of time and at different times of the day can offer a wider perspective as their strengths and needs may fluctuate, and a one-off assessment only pro-vides a snapshot.

Whilst measuring outcomes may help in monitoring and reassessing a person's occupational strengths and needs, this requires creative approaches and eliminating assumptions. Despite living with advanced dementia, a person can still have a goal that is based on their current strengths and needs. For example, a goal may be to identify a wider range of purposeful leisure occupations for everyday use, or to introduce a sensory approach to eating to enhance pleasure, stimulation, social connectedness and improve nutrition. Outcomes may also focus on family members and staff, supporting them to increase the person's autonomy during self-care tasks (Snow 2019), and to share occupational ways of communicating, such as through movement/dance and music/singing. It is important to note that many outcomes may happen 'in the moment' and can easily be overlooked or even invalidated.

Exploration of current evidence-based interventions

At the time of writing this chapter, the empirical research about occupation for people living with advanced dementia is sparse. Research studies are likely to be small-scale, with few participants who have reached the advanced stage of dementia, possibly attributable to the considerable ethical and design-based challenges for researching with this group of people. The small-scale interventions that do exist may offer a positive experience for the person with advanced dementia. These include music, experiences such as multisensory environments and complementary therapies, and object-centred activities using dolls and animal-assisted interventions (Brown *et al.* 2020). Recent innovations include the use of digital technology and enriched multisensory activities.

Small-scale or one-to-one interaction is most effective and supportive during this period (Stacpoole *et al.* 2017), combined with a focus on occupations that appeal to the senses and the natural movements, reactions and responses of the body (Brown *et al.* 2020). Music is an example, which is easily accessed, even in advanced dementia, with the potential to elicit a range of emotions, memories and responses (Mercadel-Brotons 2019). There is some evidence that music can reduce distress, improve communication and interaction (Mercadel-Brotons 2019) and enhance understanding of communication by caregivers (Wood 2019). There are many ways to introduce music to the person, their family and caregivers, such as personalized song lists, singing along with others and music therapy. However, choice is important, and it cannot be taken for granted that the person enjoys music, or any other occupation.

Multisensory interventions, for example Namaste Care, and complementary approaches using massage, reflexology and aromatherapy, have a shared focus on sensory and bodily involvement to achieve wellbeing, stimulating the senses to increase connections with others, and induce a tranquil and relaxed state. Namaste Care is a sensory, psychosocial activity that is intended to enhance the quality of life for people with advanced dementia. In the care home setting it has been shown to not only positively influence the wellbeing of the person with advanced dementia, but also their family and staff (Stacpoole *et al.* 2017). Complementary therapies are often less available in advanced dementia, however, mainly due to issues regarding the person's ability to consent. Despite this, a recent study applying aromatherapy, massage and reflexology techniques within a needs-led, individualized approach showed reduced distress for people with advanced dementia (Mitchell *et al.* 2020).

Sensory and comforting experiences can be stimulated in doll-focused activities using lifelike baby dolls that can be weighted and formed to look similar to a real baby. However, special care and planning must be implemented when considering and applying this type of intervention as the use of dolls can be controversial and seen as patronizing and childish. In practice, there may be challenges as the person may take ownership of the doll, which can create interpersonal tensions when others touch the doll. In addition, families may not understand the use of dolls as an occupation, and may feel apprehensive of their use, so communication and collaboration with families is essential. The person living with advanced dementia can also become upset if they believe the doll is a real child and feel unable to look after it; it is therefore important not just to assess, but also to reassess and work as a team to identify and evaluate the intervention. On the other hand, dolls can be soothing and calming, bringing a rich embodied experience for some people who will rock and pat the doll (Braden and Gasper 2015). Care should be taken to ensure a sensitive and comprehensive assessment is completed as some older people have experiences in their youth concerning babies that they may not have shared with family. By having the person reach for the doll rather than presenting or placing the doll in their arms, you will offer them the choice and the opportunity not to engage. Good team communication with clear protocols and regular review can help the decision as to if or when doll therapy can be used successfully.

Increasingly, animal-assisted occupations have evolved and developed for people who are in the earlier stages of dementia, with recent studies evaluating the impact of dementia assistance dogs (see Ritchie *et al.* 2019). As with all interventions it is vital to know about the person's experience and reaction to animals in their past, as some people may dislike animals or feel scared of them. It is also important to consider infection control processes, as with any intervention.

Digital approaches include the use of interactive devices that use lighting animations projected onto a table or bed and images that move in response to the person's movements, no matter how slight. These are novel, and more evidence is needed about their impact, specifically with people with advanced dementia (Bruil *et al.* 2018). Recent work is developing on the use of these digital interventions, bringing together multisensory experiences in a digital environment.

Despite these examples, evidence regarding interventions for people with advanced dementia remains sparse, with most of the research studies set in care homes. This increases the urgency of translating these studies into care-at-home with families. In the meantime, in practice, choice is a key concern, and knowledge about the person's past and current preferences and previous experiences is essential when contemplating what might prove meaningful to them. For the practitioners and families who provide the activity, there is an ongoing need to maintain a positive attitude and continually build knowledge for a positive approach to occupation in advanced dementia.

Sensory, embodied and creative approaches

The way we see a person with advanced dementia affects what we do and how we do it – our view of the person can either open up meaningful opportunities or shut them off. We will now introduce three different perspectives of advanced dementia to illustrate this point – a cognitive view, a linguistic interpretation and an embodied, creative and sensory understanding.

If we view a person through a cognitive lens, such as their ability to recall and remember things, to plan and to sequence, the person with advanced dementia is at risk of becoming demoralized, dehumanized and objectified, leading to occupational injustice (Whalley Hammell and Beagan 2017), contributing to inequality, judgement and stigma. Similarly, judging a person on their linguistic skills is not helpful to someone with advanced dementia. They may still be able to have a conversation, but the content may be incoherent to the listener, or they may only communicate through sounds and/or through bodily movements and facial expressions. We need to learn how to listen in different ways and adapt our own way of communicating, for example by tuning in to the way the person uses their voice rather than the rationality of the content (Wood 2019).

A more holistic and empathic approach is to use embodied, creative and sensory methods to uncover opportunities for 'doing, being, belonging and becoming' (Wilcock and Hocking 2015, p.147) for people living with advanced dementia. Kontos's (2005, p.556) 'embodied selfhood' encompasses the person's instinctive way of being and doing, paying attention to how they use and move their body. Kontos is one of the founders of the Reimagining Dementia coalition, working creatively to rethink and redefine dementia through exploratory drama, dance, expression, music and voice, in collaboration with a wider international team that actively includes people living with dementia. These examples empower people living with advanced dementia and their loved ones and caregivers, offering creative, occupational and social opportunities.

Creativity fits well with an occupational perspective, as it can be applied to everyday activities and tasks, using innovative ways to adapt the routine and the mundane, with the possibility of offering people with advanced dementia, their family members and caregivers more opportunities for meaningful connection. Occupations in Killick and Craig's (2012) book *Creativity and Communication in Persons with Dementia* can be easily adapted to suit the strengths of many people living with advanced dementia. They include creating a multisensory and 'textured environment' (p.114), which may involve holding and playing with coloured balls of wool, clay or paint to stimulate the senses and enrich activities.

The way you and others see people with advanced dementia is important as it affects how you interact with them, the choices and opportunities you offer, the occupations they engage in, and in turn, their wellbeing and quality of life. We encourage you to try different approaches depending on the person and their social and physical environment, and not to be discouraged if something turns out differently than expected. What works one day may not work the next, so flexibility and a co-creative approach is key, alongside continually reflecting on what worked and what could have been done differently.

Conclusion

The purpose of this chapter was to offer the reader a flavour of the potential occupational needs of people living with advanced dementia, with the intention of increasing awareness and understanding. We have outlined an array of complex needs and provided an occupational perspective of advanced dementia. The possible approaches to assessment, interventions and measuring outcomes have hopefully provided you with an initial understanding of current occupational therapy practice in this area. The take-home message is to think creatively and flexibly when working with people living with advanced dementia, their families and your colleagues. Innovative, strengths-focused, person-centred and relationship-centred approaches are vital to improve collaborative practice, and ultimately enhance the daily lives of people with advanced dementia.

Reflective questions

Reflect now on the role of creative approaches in advanced dementia, using music as an example. There is a range of online music-based interventions, and you may wish to access these to inspire and guide you when considering the following:

1. What impact might familiar or favourite music have on the person?
2. Which occupational approaches could compensate for sensory and dementia-related changes when engaging with music?
3. How might these examples of available resources be used to involve families?

Consider these questions in relation to two other creative occupations from this chapter.

References

Braden, B.A. and Gaspar, P.M. (2015) 'Implementation of a baby doll therapy protocol for people with dementia: Innovative practice.' *Dementia 14*, 5, 696–706.

Brown, M., Mitchell, B., Quinn, S., Boyd, A. and Tolson, D. (2020) 'Introduction to living with advanced dementia series.' *Nursing Older People 32*, 3, 12–16.

Bruil, L., Adriaansen, M., Groothuis, J. and Bossema, E. (2018) 'Quality of life of nursing home residents with dementia before, during and after playing with a magic table.' *Tijdschrift voor gerontologie en geriatrie 49*, 2, 72–80.

Cooper, J.R., Parkinson, S., de las Heras de Pablo, C.G., Shute, R., Melton, J. and Forsyth, K. (2014) *A User's Manual for the Model of Human Occupation Exploratory Level Outcome Ratings (MOHO-ExpLOR)*, Version 1.0. Edinburgh: Queen Margaret University.

Ellis, M. and Astell, A. (2017) 'Communicating with people living with dementia who are nonverbal: The creation of adaptive interaction.' *PLOS ONE 12*, 8, 1–21.

Holmerova, I., Waugh, A., MacRae, R., Veprkova, R., *et al.* (2016) *Dementia Palliare Best Practice Statement*. European Commission, University of the West of Scotland.

Jack-Waugh, A., Henderson, J., Sharp, B., Holland, S. and Brown, M. (2020) 'Delivering personal care for people with advanced dementia.' *Nursing Older People 32*, 5, 1–15.

Killick, J. and Craig, C. (2012) *Creativity and Communication in Persons with Dementia – A Practical Guide*. London: Jessica Kingsley Publishers.

Kontos, P. (2005) 'Embodied selfhood in Alzheimer's disease: Rethinking person-centred care.' *Dementia 4*, 4, 553–570.

Mercadel-Brotons, M. (2019) 'Music Interventions for Advanced Dementia: Needs and Clinical Interventions Identified from a Narrative Synthesis Review.' In A. Baird, S. Garrido and J. Tamplin (eds) *Music and Dementia: From Cognition to Therapy* (pp.242–268). Oxford: Oxford University Press.

Mitchell, B., Jackson, G.A., Sharp, B. and Tolson, D. (2020) 'Complementary therapy for advanced dementia palliation in nursing homes.' *Journal of Integrated Care 28*, 4, 419–432. https://doi.org/10.1108/JICA-02-2020-0009

Perrin, T., May, H. and Anderson, E. (2008) *Wellbeing in Dementia: An Occupational Approach for Therapists and Carers* (2nd edn). Edinburgh: Churchill Livingstone.

Pool, J. (2012) *The Pool Activity Level (PAL) Instrument for Occupational Profiling: A Practical Resource for Carers of People with Cognitive Impairment* (4th edn). London and Philadelphia, PA: Jessica Kingsley Publishers.

Ritchie, L., Quinn, S., Tolson, D., Jenkins, N. and Sharp, B. (2019) 'Exposing the mechanisms underlying successful animal assisted interventions for people with dementia: A realistic evaluation of the Dementia Dog Project.' *Dementia 20*, 1. https://doi.org/10.1177/1471301219864505

SCIE (Social Care Institute for Excellence) (2014) 'Living with dementia.' London: SCIE. Accessed on 14/09/2021 at www.youtube.com/watch?v=loksPQ7Q8tM

Snow, T. (2019) 'How to help a person living with dementia brush their teeth.' Accessed on 14/09/2021 at www.youtube.com/watch?v=6gLrH8mioCw&t=15s

Souyave, J., Treadway, C., Fennell, J. and Walters, A. (2019) 'Designing Folding Interventions for Positive Moments.' In K. Neidderer, G. Ludden, R. Cain and C. Wölfel (eds)

Proceedings of the MinD International Conference: Designing with and for People with Dementia: Wellbeing Happiness and Empowerment (pp.57–68). Dresden: TUD Press.

Stacpoole, M., Hockley, J., Thompsell, A., Simard, J. and Volicer, L. (2017) 'Implementing the Namaste Care program for residents with advanced dementia: Exploring the perceptions of families and staff in UK care homes.' *Annals of Palliative Medicine* 6, 4, 327–339.

Whalley Hammell, K.R. and Beagan, B. (2017) 'Occupational injustice: A critique.' *Canadian Journal of Occupational Therapy 84*, 1, 58–68.

Wilcock, A. and Hocking, C. (2015) *An Occupational Perspective of Health* (3rd edn). Thorofare, NJ: SLACK Incorporated.

Wood, S. (2019) 'Beyond Messiaen's birds: The post-verbal world of dementia.' *Medical Humanities 46*, 73–83.

CHAPTER 10

The Three 'C's' of Curricula Redesign

Conversations, Courage and Change in Dementia Education

Fiona Maclean, Michelle Elliot and Elaine Hunter

Learning outcomes

By the end of this chapter, you will have the opportunity to:

▸ Understand the wider context reflecting a need for change in how enhanced dementia awareness is taught across pre- and post-registration occupational therapy education at one university in the UK

▸ Appraise the ways learning can be widened to include occupational therapy internships that can help to construct a professional narrative supportive of a rights-based approach to dementia practice

▸ Inspire future-focused conversations that encourage occupational therapy learners to evolve and become agents of change in practice.

Introduction

We know occupational therapists will likely meet someone living with dementia at some point in their professional or personal lives, and for some, working with people living with dementia will be the prime focus of their role. This likelihood is influenced by the increasing scale of the health and social needs of those living with dementia. For example, in Scotland it is estimated that 90,000 people live with a diagnosis of dementia (Alzheimer Scotland 2021), and approximately 50 million people globally (WHO 2020).

The extent to which dementia impacts people, families and their communities therefore influenced a conversation that took place in 2012 between two authors (and occupational therapists) of this chapter: Fiona, an academic at a higher education institute, and Elaine, a national consultant allied health professional with Scotland's leading dementia charity, Alzheimer Scotland. This conversation recognized the important role and potential contribution of both the existing and future allied health professions (AHP) workforce to act as agents of change, to begin to shift practice in dementia towards a rights-based approach. However, to do so would mean, in part, widening access to AHP educational opportunities with the aim of integrating new and evolving evidence in, for example, brain health and the right to rehabilitation in everyday practice.

There already exist several initiatives that aim to support occupational therapists in becoming skilled and confident when working with people living with dementia (Jack-Waugh, Ritchie and MacRae 2018; Smith et al. 2019). Yet evidence indicates that knowledge of dementia in the AHP workforce could be enhanced (Lawler et al. 2020). This informed our view that partnership working in dementia education is key – to enable practitioners, graduates and students of occupational therapy to further grow their confidence in learning about and working with people living with dementia. Consequently, the work and perspectives presented here reflect one example of a partnership that developed between Scotland's leading dementia charity, Alzheimer Scotland, and pre- and post-registration occupational therapy education delivered by Queen Margaret University, Edinburgh.

This chapter begins with an outline of the policy context, underpinned by a human rights-based approach, which influenced conversations between Alzheimer Scotland and members of the occupational therapy teaching team at Queen Margaret University. These conversations supported identification of the qualities of educational change that were needed, including the value and importance of use of language, and reciprocity of learning between students of occupational therapy and people with lived experience of dementia. Examples of how educational change has been implemented are illustrated, including an outline of the creation of an occupational therapy internship programme that aims to bridge learning and teaching between students of occupational therapy with the voices and experiences of people living with dementia.

Context-shaping conversations

Dementia as a global health concern has gradually been recognized, with an emphasis on the need to support the rights of people living with dementia (Alzheimer's Disease International 2020). This included the creation of the Glasgow Declaration, which sought to commit all members of Alzheimer Europe to affirm every person living with dementia has:

- The right to a timely diagnosis
- The right to access quality post-diagnostic support
- The right to person centred, coordinated, quality care throughout their illness
- The right to equitable access to treatments and therapeutic interventions
- The right to be respected as an individual in their community. (Alzheimer Europe 2014)

This Declaration informed how European policy should respond, by supporting the design of tailored national Dementia Strategies targeting the nuances of population need, whilst also reflecting commonality influenced by the principles of a rights-based approach. The translation and adoption of an explicitly rights-based approach in practice, as well as in policy, was an inevitable outcome from this Declaration.

For allied health professionals, there was, and still is, a lack of published evidence or debate that directly addresses what a rights-based approach looks like when working with people living with dementia, their families and caregivers. Nevertheless, Scotland was one of the first nations to publish an evidence-based AHP dementia policy, *Connecting People, Connecting Support* (Alzheimer Scotland 2017, 2020). This policy intended to strategically encourage, prompt and transform practice, including the profession of occupational therapy, towards a rights-based approach. To mobilize implementation and integration of this policy with practice, partnership working with educational institutions was recognized as essential, and in particular, the transformative role education can play to grow and support a skilled and confident occupational therapy workforce in dementia.

Hocking and Ness (2005) were amongst the first to emphasize the point that there is a need for occupational therapy education to understand, be relevant and responsive to the local health and social needs of communities and populations. This ongoing challenge means professional education must consistently strive to enhance diversity, not only in what learners are taught, but also how they are taught. For graduates and the profession to continue to be effective, learning and teaching connected to the contribution of occupational therapy in dementia needs to be iteratively refreshed.

This wider context directed and informed the beginning of an ongoing process to redesign how professional dementia education at Queen Margaret University was taught. This necessitated courage to value, invest in and progress the emergence of a trusting strategic partnership between occupational therapy educators and Alzheimer Scotland. The vision was to establish an educational partnership that could reimagine what and how innovations in learning and teaching could evolve, with the intent of leading change. Specifically, it was to facilitate occupational therapy students to become agents of change, confident in dementia practice, with the goal of achieving better outcomes for people living with dementia, their families and caregivers.

Initially, what we taught at Queen Margaret University needed to advance understanding and consideration of dementia 'care', which historically could view people with dementia as a uniform group of care recipients. Instead, as Bartlett and O'Connor (2010) have suggested, people living with dementia represent a diverse group of people, with unique personal experiences, culture(s), networks of support and social positions. To work in partnership with people living with dementia we needed to value, understand and document their unique experiences and beliefs. This understanding influenced how we wanted occupational therapy dementia education to evolve, recognizing that teaching and learning are not synonymous. Not all learning is immediately or consciously experienced as transformative, just as learning does not exclusively occur in designated 'education' settings, such as university classrooms or practice contexts. We aspired to bridge and change conversations within classrooms and communities, to engage with curiosity and criticality, and to work to establish reciprocity of learning from and with people living with dementia. It was this vision that was both transformational and tangible, and that will be discussed in greater detail in subsequent sections.

Qualities of courage

Across the life course, we experience many different spaces and places of and for learning. The desire of many pre- and post-registration AHP students is to learn 'how to' – how to work with individuals living with dementia; how to work in an occupation-, person-centred, holistic manner; and how to incorporate conceptual models and published evidence into treatment processes. Our experiences working with pre-registration students reflected that experiential, practice-based learning within immersive contexts beyond university classrooms was often perceived to be richer or more 'relevant' than the theory and academic-focused learning processes.

Despite the wording, learning 'how to' is often reduced to pragmatic education about 'what to do'. The complexity of everyday life and the diversity of people and experiences do not neatly or ethically align with such a reductionist approach. What and how we learn is informed by what and how we are taught, as well as how and in what ways we are open to the sources of knowledge around us.

Pedagogical approaches over the years have shifted away from passive absorption of wisdom from a learned scholar at the front of a lecture theatre, although this is still likely to be found in higher education. Active processes of engagement inclusive of discussion, reflection and debate underpin the development of critical thinking and the potential for transformative learning (Mezirow 2018). The adoption of a worldview where multiple perspectives are valued, where a diversity of experiences is presented, and whereby expertise is collectively shared, all reflect the process of widening formal learning spaces. For conversations to facilitate change, conversations themselves need to change, and change requires courage. Within our work, this courage was to think constructively and critically about existing processes of education, and how these could be grown to include the voice(s) of people living with dementia, their families and caregivers.

This iterative process of diversifying conversations and perspectives of learning about dementia, framed by the courage to influence change, led to innovation to create the first paid Alzheimer Scotland/Santander Universities UK occupational therapy internship programme (Maclean, Elliot and Hunter 2019). Considered in further detail later in this chapter, the internship programme ran over a period of seven years. Twelve occupational therapy interns (pre- and post-registration students, including recent graduates of Queen Margaret University) undertook projects predominantly in partnership with the Scottish Dementia Working Group (SDWG; see Chapter 1). Membership of this group requires a diagnosis of dementia. In the work we completed with the SDWG, we ensured that 'case studies' were neither paper exercises nor theoretically conceptualized. Instead, we challenged our beliefs and the sources of our knowledge (Berg, Philipp and Taff 2019) through curriculum and conversations facilitated and informed by people living with dementia and their families. This allowed interns to work in partnership with people living with dementia to co-create and co-design projects, and therefore generate outcomes of relevance to the SDWG.

Learning from these collaborations, we contend that the language and imagery associated with dementia in education must be critically considered, within the casual conversations we have, the media we consume and the professional discourse we contribute to. For example, images found on different internet search engines infer that an individual with dementia is becoming invisible, with cognitive capacity floating away like leaves on a tree. A focus on symptomology and deficits related to dementia fails to retain the humanity and wider narrative of a person living with dementia and their interests, capacity and meaningful occupations. A person's love of walking may become pathologized when that same person receives a diagnosis of dementia. 'They' might be at risk of 'wandering'.

The homogeneity of experiences of people living with dementia is often reflected in headlines or sound bites using the language of 'suffering' or 'victims'. As a profession, we need to work hard to challenge and change the conversation, and this begins with greater awareness of the words we use. Swaffer (2014), an Australian writer, activist and woman living with dementia, put forward that call to action, cautioning that a failure to do so is a human rights violation.

Disempowering language becomes appropriated into common discourse, normalizing stereotypes, stigma and discrimination. Words and language also hold culturally and socially constructed meaning; when we change how we speak, we must ensure the intention of our words is also revised. Moreover, the contexts in which we speak, listen, share and engage – our learning spaces – also challenge us to consider who 'holds' the knowledge, the power and the expertise within the conversations that are generated within the spaces. We also find that there has been a need to design 'dementia language' guidelines (Dementia Australia 2018), noting the words we use to talk about dementia can have a significant impact on how people with dementia are viewed and treated in our communities. The use of language, reciprocity of learning and recognizing the need to bridge learning and teaching between communities were all qualities that framed our courage to reshape and inform the changes we needed to make in occupational therapy dementia education.

Changes in action

As highlighted earlier in this chapter, the value and importance of partnership working was regarded as crucial to developing positive approaches to learning and teaching in dementia education. Building on an understanding of the need to bridge between communities and widen educational spaces beyond the classroom, Alzheimer Scotland and Queen Margaret University developed an occupational therapy internship programme, supported by the SDWG. Whilst internships are variously defined across the literature, they typically involve students or recent graduates (usually within two years of degree completion) undertaking a set period of work with an employer, in an area of specialism, which connects to their career aspirations. In this case, the internship programme provided an opportunity to co-create projects designed to support the aims of the SDWG – to promote and raise awareness of dementia amongst health, social care and related professions, including the wider public, for example.

The responsibility to raise awareness of dementia was embedded throughout the application process. Applicants to the internship programme were all guaranteed an interview, and all received feedback on their performance, including ways their professional interest in dementia might continue to grow. The decision to offer an interview at the application stage to all was also designed to give applicants an equal opportunity to succeed, in tandem progressing their skills related to their employability for the future.

The benefits to the employer of the internship programme, in this case Alzheimer Scotland, were to help infuse fresh perspectives and new ideas into the team. Additionally, it promoted specialized careers in dementia practice as a destination of choice for new graduates, to help support a future talented workforce. In turn, the internship partnership helped to update and refresh university curricula for all occupational therapy learners to benefit from.

Consequently, the internship programme consisted of a three-way partnership between the intern (an occupational therapy pre- or post-registration student or recent graduate), Queen Margaret University and the internship 'host' or employer (SDWG and Alzheimer Scotland), as highlighted in Figure 10.1.

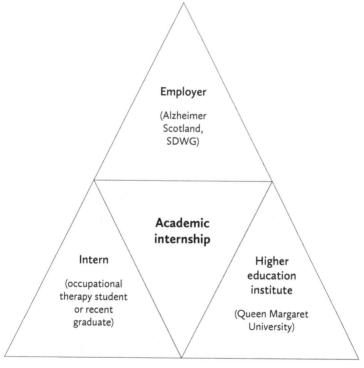

Figure 10.1. A three-way academic internship partnership

The underpinning ethos of the internship programme evolved over time, and ultimately sought to:

- Raise wider awareness of the rights of people diagnosed with dementia to engage in occupations identified by the person as important to their health and wellbeing, to support their right to continue to live well with dementia
- Diversify the ways through which occupational therapy education can embrace, extend and include wider learning opportunities for occupational therapy students, beyond practice education, to enhance knowledge and understanding of working with people living with dementia, their families and caregiver(s)
- Proactively encourage occupational therapy students and recent graduates to pursue specialized career paths in dementia practice, underpinned by enhanced knowledge
- Empower future therapists to work in partnership with people living with dementia and their caregivers, at all points from diagnosis, and to challenge stigma by working with, and learning from, people with lived experience, in this case, members of the SDWG.

As a result, projects created were designed to bring people together. The projects undertaken by interns helped to widen education to allow people living with dementia to directly influence pre- and post-graduate occupational therapy learning. This included the ways in which teaching content was identified and prioritized by people living with dementia and integrated as part of curriculum redesign.

For example, an initial internship project asked members of the SDWG, 'What is important to me?' This question was asked because it was essential to understand what people living with dementia prioritized as important, so this could become core to learning and teaching content. It also helped to 'trial' a simple question that any occupational therapist could ask at any time and in any practice setting when working with someone with dementia or, indeed, any community of people. The humanity of responses was striking, all of which emphasized the need to promote healthy, positive and respectful relationships in practice, the foundation of adopting a rights-based approach. Two of the initial responses to 'What is important to me?' included:

> To be heard. To be listened to. To be treated with dignity and respect. To be treated the same as we treat anyone else.

> To challenge stigma and that we all work together to respect each other.

Two further projects sought to develop and promote self-management resources. In partnership with the SDWG two peer-to-peer resources for people recently diagnosed with dementia were created and published. This involved asking members of the SDWG 'What are your top tips to living well with dementia?' and 'What is the one thing you wish you had been told from somebody with dementia after being diagnosed?'

Answers led to the creation of two self-management resources available on the SDWG website. One offers a range of practical tips that can be used to live well with dementia, from those with lived experience. The second co-designed booklet offers advice on what members of the SDWG found useful when receiving a diagnosis of dementia. Both questions led to the collation of booklets, to be shared more widely with people who are living with dementia.

This vision to widen educational spaces to diversify the contexts where learning occurred also led to the integration of third sector AHP practice placements, based within the policy and research team at Alzheimer Scotland. The important and critical role of practice-based learning for future ideas and values of occupational therapists is well documented, as are the opportunities for diverse placements (Clarke and Thornton 2014; Clarke *et al.* 2015). However, little is written about the opportunities that exist in working directly with the third sector as an important lever of change for our future workforce – in this case, how and in what way a human rights-based approach to dementia, as adopted by Alzheimer Scotland, can influence, inform and potentially change the way(s) in which occupational therapy learners view dementia. Profiling an understanding of the pivotal role third sector practice-based learning can offer connected to the Scottish Government's drive towards health and social care integration is reflected by Henry Simmons, chief executive of Alzheimer Scotland:

When you come (as an occupational therapy student) you get this experience, you see the whole thing, hearing about what people are fundraising for, hearing about what we are campaigning for, hearing what people are engaged in for their challenges and issues and perhaps most importantly, to get a chance to sit down and listen to people. (Simmons 2014)

Diversifying educational spaces to include an occupational therapy internship programme and third sector practice-based learning relied on the involvement and connections with hitherto 'unknown' communities, such as the SDWG, to broaden the lens of where learning was possible. In so doing, this sharing, or mutuality of learning, has led to positive, dynamic and interactive relationships, which has inspired changes in how interns act and think. It offers the possibility to reshape their professional practice and, indeed, influence those around them. For example, occupational therapy interns who worked with members of the SDWG have reflexively acknowledged:

The internship with Alzheimer Scotland has allowed me to understand and advocate for the rights of people living with dementia.

These experiences of learning together have stayed with me and positively impact my day-to-day working life as an occupational therapist, post the internship, with people living with dementia in an array of settings.

I have learned the importance to make no assumptions, remove judgements, be patient and kind.

Similarly, members of the SDWG who worked with the occupational therapy interns highlighted mutuality of learning:

They find out things from us, but we're learning just as much from them – that stands out.

Normally younger people and older people, they are that far apart, but when they [interns] start working with us, we're as close as that. We're very close together – that's the beauty of the internship.

Conclusion

This chapter has concentrated on the importance of coming together through valuing partnerships that can embrace conversations to identify the qualities of courage needed to positively navigate towards a refreshed future direction of change in occupational therapy dementia education. At its very best, education and lifelong learning can support occupational therapists at various stages of their career to become the agents of change needed in practice to enhance, in this case, outcomes for people living with dementia and their caregivers. The phrase 'agents of change' can appear glib, or even vague, when trying to understand what and how we strive towards in practice. In our partnerships and learning processes, we recognize how knowledge and action, policy and practice, conversations and curiosity, are dynamic. Changes to one might change the other. To be an 'agent' is to consider oneself 'agentic' – taking and seeking action. Across the profession we each hold this responsibility, regardless of context.

Therefore, when working with people living with dementia and their caregivers, your knowledge, experience and expertise influencing what you do and how you do it counts. This includes the language that you use, alongside your ability to listen and respect diverse views and perspectives, recognizing the heterogeneity of experience(s) prevalent when working with people living with dementia. We must also be aware we often do not know the answer. However, through valuing evidence in all its forms, including reciprocity of learning and in holding an aspiration to build and advance bridges between education, learners, third sector partners and, most importantly, the experts by experience, we will enhance the possibility of creating meaningful change in how we deliver our services. Most importantly, by building on and iteratively evolving how we think about and work in partnership, we will become far better equipped as a profession to effectively advocate for the rights of people living with dementia as equal citizens, as part of our communities.

Reflective questions

1. In your daily life, how do you apply a critical lens to what you hear, read or share about people living with dementia?

2. What are your values and beliefs when you imagine yourself working with people living with dementia?

3. If you were to engage in the process of curriculum development related to dementia in your programme of study, how would you propose inviting the perspectives of people living with dementia, their caregivers and their family members? What could be expanded on in your current programme or service?

References

Alzheimer Europe (2014) *Glasgow Declaration 2014.* Luxembourg: Alzheimer Europe. Accessed on 01/04/2021 at www.alzheimer-europe.org/policy/campaign/glasgow-declaration-2014

Alzheimer Scotland (2017) *Connecting People, Connecting Support: Transforming the Allied Health Professionals' Contribution to Supporting People Living with Dementia in Scotland, 2017–2020.* Edinburgh: Alzheimer Scotland. Accessed on 06/05/2021 at www.alzscot.org/sites/default/files/images/0002/9408/AHP_Report_2017_Web.pdf

Alzheimer Scotland (2020) *Connecting People, Connecting Support in Action: An Impact Report on Transforming the Allied Health Professions Contribution to Supporting People Living with Dementia in Scotland.* Edinburgh: Alzheimer Scotland. Accessed on 25/04/2022 at www.alzscot.org/sites/default/files/2020-03/Connecting%20People%20Connecting%20Support%20in%20action%20report.pdf

Alzheimer Scotland (2021) 'Statistics.' Edinburgh: Alzheimer Scotland. Accessed on 01/04/2021 at www.alzscot.org/our-work/campaigning-for-change/scotlands-national-dementia-strategy/statistics

Alzheimer's Disease International (2020) 'Human rights.' London: Alzheimer's Disease International. Accessed on 01/04/2021 at www.alzint.org/what-we-do/policy/human-rights

Bartlett, R. and O'Connor, D. (2010) *Broadening the Dementia Debate towards Social Citizenship.* Bristol: Policy Press.

Berg, C., Philipp, R. and Taff, S.D. (2019) 'Critical thinking and transformational learning: Using case studies as narrative frameworks for threshold concepts.' *Journal of Occupational Therapy Education 3*, 3. https://doi.org/10.26681/jote.2019.030313

Clarke, C., Martin, M., de Visser, R. and Sadlo, G. (2015) 'Sustaining professional identity in practice following role-emerging placements: Opportunities and challenges for occupational therapists.' *British Journal of Occupational Therapy 78*, 1, 42–50.

Clarke, M. and Thornton, J. (2014) 'Using appreciative inquiry to explore the potential of enhanced practice education opportunities.' *British Journal of Occupational Therapy 77*, 9, 475–487.

Dementia Australia (2018) *Dementia Language Guidelines.* Accessed on 30/03/2021 at www.dementia.org.au/sites/default/files/resources/dementia-language-guidelines.pdf

Hocking, C. and Ness, N.E. (2005) 'Professional Education in Context.' In G. Whiteford and V. Wright-St Clair (eds) *Occupation and Practice in Context* (pp.3–15). London: Elsevier Churchill Livingstone.

Jack-Waugh, A., Ritchie, L. and MacRae, R. (2018) 'Assessing the educational impact of the dementia champions programme in Scotland: Implications for evaluating professional dementia education.' *Nurse Education Today 71*, 205–210.

Lawler, K., Kitsos, A., Bindoff, A.D., Callisaya, M.L., Eccleston, C.E.A. and Doherty, K.V. (2020) 'Room for improvement: An online survey of allied health professionals' dementia knowledge.' *Australasian Journal on Ageing 40*, 2, 195–201.

Maclean, F., Elliot, M.L. and Hunter, E. (2019) 'A pathway to success.' *OTnews 27*, 3, 30–32.

Mezirow, J. (2018) 'Transformative Learning Theory.' In K. Illeris (ed.) *Contemporary Theories of Learning: Learning Theorists...in Their Own Words* (2nd edn, pp.114–128). Abingdon: Routledge.

Simmons, H. (2014) 'Allied heath professional students' experiences of placements within Alzheimer Scotland.' Accessed on 15/07/2021 at https://vimeo.com/129880962

Smith, S., Parveen, S., Sass, C., Drury, M., Oyebode, J.R. and Surr, C.A. (2019) 'An audit of dementia education and training in UK health and social care: A comparison with national benchmark standards.' *BMC Health Services Research 19*. Accessed on 06/07/2021 at https://bmchealthservres.biomedcentral.com/articles/10.1186/s12913-019-4510-6

Swaffer, K. (2014) 'Dementia: Stigma, language, and dementia-friendly.' *Dementia 13*, 6, 709–716.

WHO (World Health Organization) (2021) 'Dementia.' Fact sheets, 2 September. Accessed on 25/11/2021 at www.who.int/news-room/fact-sheets/detail/dementia

OCCUPATION

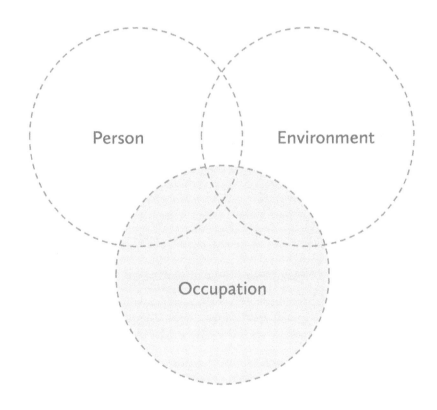

Occupation, Social Participation and Rights-Based Practice in South West England

Examining Health and Wellbeing for People with Dementia through a Community Lens

Lyn Westcott and Kimberley Crocker-White

Learning outcomes

By the end of this chapter, you will have the opportunity to:

▸ Reflect on occupational justice to promote health and wellbeing for people living with dementia, their families and caregivers in community settings
▸ Identify factors that can promote or impede social justice, human rights and personhood for people living with dementia
▸ Identify how the need for social participation through occupation may change through a person's unique dementia journey
▸ Consider capacity and consent in relation to people with dementia having access to meaningful occupations in community settings.

Introduction

The theory guiding occupational therapy practice clearly highlights that people are not only occupational beings, but are also embedded in a social or interpersonal world where their personhood is shaped, affirmed and provided with meaning. Social participation is linked with wellbeing, maintaining and improving personal health. Models of occupational therapy highlight the importance of social environments as vital components in theoretical frameworks to explain people's experiences of occupation (Fisher, Parkinson and Haglund 2017; Iwama 2006). Social environments might suggest a static state surrounding a person. Instead, it is helpful to see social environments as dynamic, ever-changing circumstances. This includes other people and what they do, as well as the culture that guides their actions. Social environments also include broader dimensions – things people may feel they have less agency to challenge or change, such as legislation and policy that influences services offered.

The theory of occupational science upholds that people have a need to participate in their social environments, and an inability to do this leads to occupational deprivation (Whiteford 2000), which is part of a wider agenda of occupational justice for everyone (Townsend and Wilcock 2004). So, denial of occupational participation in a social world can be detrimental to both a person's and a community's health and wellbeing, in addition to impacting on individual rights for members of society (Wilcock and Hocking 2015). It is not only a health issue but also one of justice and equality of opportunity. If this is the case, occupational therapists and the services where they work should enable social participation for people using those services and their caregivers.

This chapter explores these issues largely from the context of community settings (with anonymised examples based broadly on experience), illustrating a realistic view of people living with dementia at different stages of progression and receiving supportive occupational therapy interventions. It also outlines some considerations of capacity in terms of community settings, as this can influence how occupational therapists work with people living with dementia. It is informed by occupational therapy practice in South West England, a largely rural and coastal area popular amongst retirees, many remote from nuclear family networks, presenting extra challenges during ageing, including living with dementia. Although it is acknowledged that dementia can begin at a younger age, South West England is recognized as having a higher-than-average UK population over 65 years, thus leading to higher incidences of dementia (ONS 2021).

Occupational justice, health and wellbeing for people living with dementia and their families and carers in community settings

The concept of occupational justice identifies that participation should reinforce human health by means of access to social opportunities and resources (Townsend and Wilcock 2004). Subsequently, occupational injustices occur when participation in occupations is restricted, marginalized and/or devalued, and the impact is recognized as severe and long-lasting (Laliberte Rudman 2012). The context and environment surrounding participation directly influences an individual's ability to thrive, a notion that is imperative for people with dementia and their caregivers, and a key concern for occupational therapists working in community settings.

Social participation is a prominent influence on quality of life and wellbeing for all older people (Dawson-Townsend 2019), reaffirming self-concept and maintaining personal identity and autonomy. In an occupationally just social environment, people living with dementia would have the right to engage and experience social inclusion, a point seen as positively impacting on health and wellbeing by Whalley Hammell (2013). Recent changes in the UK's community practice have echoed the prominent shift from a medical-focused care environment, opening the door for occupational therapy and the application of occupation within everyday settings. This enables services and practitioners to think more holistically about people they work with, being aware of their psychosocial environment and how this impacts on their wellbeing. The focus on rights-based practice, where the person is at the core, has become more prominent, actively striving for social justice for people with dementia. This notion is furthered with dementia being increasingly recognized as a disability, which has created opportunities for collaborations between people living with dementia and disability rights activists to push for social change (Kinderman *et al.* 2018). This move is aligned with the person-centred agenda advocated by occupational therapists.

People living with dementia have a fundamental right to participate in all parts of society, being valued and respected (National Dementia Action Alliance 2021). The right to a full and meaningful life does not lessen as dementia progresses; however, individuals' vulnerability to injustices may increase if their voice is not heard or valued. Health and social care professionals working with people living with dementia have both moral and ethical responsibilities to confront such injustices and advocate for those unable to do so themselves.

A reduction in social participation and engagement is linked to faster cognitive decline, changes to identity, mood and quality of life for people with dementia and their caregivers (Dawson-Townsend 2019). Personal communities structured on both informal and formal relationships support and enhance a sense of belonging and identity, whereas inclusion in peer support groups has been found to increase wellbeing (DH 2009).

One of the chapter authors (Kimberley) is involved in Memory Maintenance, a community-based, and occupation-focused group that provides weekly cognitive stimulation advice and techniques for people living with dementia. The occupational therapy-led group aims to provide a sense of social connectedness, mutual sharing and support within a familiar and inclusive environment. The group format also allows its members to share experiences and collectively problem-solve towards more positive change, both individually and as a community.

Non-pharmacological occupationally focused interventions, used in occupational therapy, are imperative in optimizing people's abilities and occupational performance, thus working to address the severity of behavioural changes and psychological symptoms of dementia. Additionally, positive effects have been found in reducing caregivers' distress as a dementia progresses, reducing their sense of burden and improving their feelings of competence (Behr and Tebb 2016).

We have noted that people living well with dementia in the community have a greater sense of wellbeing, reduced functional decline, delayed admission to care homes and improved quality of life if they engage with social and meaningful occupations.

Hollis continued jogging in his local community two years after being diagnosed with Lewy body dementia because the route was familiar to him. Both Hollis and his wife recognized that jogging could present risks, but his enjoyment outweighed these, and he has the right to take risks. He wanted to continue this routine as part of his self-care. The occupational therapist suggested Hollis wore an identity bracelet to help him feel confident in his ability to find his way home again, as he worried he might become lost. When the dementia progressed, Hollis continued walking the route with a neighbour and their dog.

> He enjoyed being outside talking with his friend about their shared
> love of motorbikes and the changes to the neighbourhood. His wife
> appreciated Hollis's continued connection with the outdoors and
> activities he enjoyed, valuing this time for her own needs.

A rights-based approach to care within the community can maintain a person's autonomy and personal identity through social participation and engagement in occupations that are valued by that individual.

Social justice, human rights and personhood

Due to the progressive nature of dementia, difficulties maintaining social participation can be experienced, compounding unmet needs and impacting on a person's health and wellbeing. Barriers to sustaining social participation in social environments can directly result from the developing condition. A randomized control trial by Kinderman *et al.* (2018), found these barriers included higher rates of anxiety and depression amongst people living with dementia. There was decreased motivation and changes to personal characteristics, including disinhibition, irritability and a focus towards the self rather than others. It is important to recognize that occupational injustices also occur when occupational choices are diminished, meaning people experience lack of control over their own lives. Such consequences are pertinent for individuals with dementia and also for family and caregivers, who themselves experience social isolation, stress and a decreased quality of life.

Kitwood (1997), in his seminal work, argued that if social attitudes and external factors were supportive and appropriate to people living with dementia, then the nature of their experiences would change for the better. However, Kinderman *et al.* (2018) highlighted that people with dementia continue to be identified amongst the most devalued and stigmatized groups, with social exclusion a common side effect. This compounds concern about the relevance of social participation in enhancing wellbeing. Stigma is not only a barrier to social participation, but it also impedes society's ability for social change required to facilitate the inclusion of people living with dementia, hence maintaining their wellbeing.

Similarly, age discrimination towards older adults can impede social justice amongst the largest population of people living with dementia

(Alzheimer's Research UK 2020). There can be a lack of mental health services for this age group, impacting on early diagnosis and lack of appropriate services. Furthermore, over 40,000 people under 65 have been diagnosed with early onset dementia in the UK (Dementia UK 2020). These individuals may also encounter discrimination, stigma and exclusion from existing dementia services, due to the focus primarily being on older adults.

Raising awareness and understanding of dementia and human rights, promoting inclusion, social participation and challenging negative stereotypes are positive methods of counteracting the negative connotations and stigma around dementia. Organizations like the Alzheimer's Society run several projects to combat stigma in general and with specific populations. Positive reporting of well-known people living with dementia in the media and their campaigning work has also helped address this, including the experiences of author Terry Pratchett and actor Barbara Windsor, who both lived at home with dementia. Caregivers can be important facilitators alongside practitioners, empowering individuals to overcome the associated stigma of dementia. Once these active approaches are being taken to reduce such stigma and discrimination, the rights of people living with dementia can be upheld and facilitated through participation and access to the meaningful occupations of daily life.

The implementation of dementia-friendly communities provides scope to promote the rights of people with dementia (Alzheimer's Society United Against Dementia 2021). This approach advocates that many barriers to participation come from the social environment not understanding or accommodating the needs of a person living with dementia. It promotes social change, through communities that reflect the needs of people with dementia in a safe and inclusive way. This means people living with dementia can continue to engage in meaningful activities as part of their communities. This type of view aligns with that of environmental adaptation, which is familiar to occupational therapists.

> Roger went into town to meet friends; however, on his return he was unable to find the correct bus time and missed the last bus home. The bus station was noisy and crowded, there were no seats

to rest on, and a new and confusing interactive screen had replaced the usual bus timetable. Roger was eventually returned home by the police after he was found walking on a busy road. The implications of this event for Roger, who has Alzheimer's disease, were that his family prevented him from going out alone, reducing his social participation and wellbeing. The occupational therapist worked with Roger and his family to safely reintroduce this meaningful activity within his weekly routine, initially accompanying him on the route and ensuring he was comfortable within the bus station environment by identifying a quieter space where he could rest and get help if needed, then employing graded goal-setting techniques to enable Roger to use the interactive screen to find his correct bus time. Furthermore, the therapist introduced the bus company to the local Dementia Friends training sessions. This provided dementia-related educational information to the bus drivers, including how to help people to live well, thus enhancing access and ease of using public transport for people living with dementia, as well as supporting Roger and his family.

Due to the geographical context within South West England, occupational injustices can occur for people with dementia. Occupational therapist practitioners must be culturally competent (Whalley Hammell 2013), understand and acknowledge that external factors, such as political infrastructure, public transport, geographical location and availability of appropriate health services, are all interdependent and impact on health status and wellbeing. In South West England this may mean working with people living in rural poverty with poor public transport and away from health or social care support structures. Interventions, as with Roger above, can positively enhance lives moving forward. Similarly, there is need to promote the active involvement of people with dementia in both research and within the formulation of local and national policies and services, considering the regional factors that impact on future care provisions. Occupational therapists can work with people to ensure they access the services they need and work with them in influencing policy development for future users (see also Chapter 7).

Occupation and social participation throughout the dementia journey

All people are unique and live in different circumstances. Everyone's life experiences, values, desires and resources available to them shape the person they are, their occupational priorities or needs and how they may meet those needs and aspirations.

People give to and receive from the social environments in which they live, physically, socially and emotionally. This process can seem interdependent in many ways, and self-sustaining. People do things together because it feeds their sense of wellbeing and belonging, prompting social participation; moreover, it helps reduce loneliness, experienced in 40 per cent of older adults (Bekhet and Zauszniewski 2012). Social participation through occupation helps a sense of belonging to a wider community of like-minded people, where your identity is also linked to skills in a given activity, for example being a gardener, or volunteering with a chosen charity that has personal meaning. For a person living with dementia, an extra layer of complexity is added to these dimensions. There may be a sense of loss, not only of giving up things that now seem too difficult, but also towards future opportunities that will be missed. Maintaining a sense of self and belonging through social participation is vital.

Cognitive changes associated with dementia mean that people living with the condition may need more support to continue social participation within the community. Occupational therapy can support people to maintain social connections and occupations that are valued and meaningful for them. Part of the participation agenda needs to respond to the changes that can occur, and may need to be reconsidered several times in someone's dementia journey. Some of the changes, such as fatigue and mobility issues, can be mitigated by pacing, timing and energy conservation, therefore saving effort for more valued occupations, such as by taking a taxi and not a bus to a valued activity. This ensures someone maintains contact with others, thus affirming their sense of self. There may also be a need for positive risk-taking inherent in person-centred working that may be uncomfortable for some practitioners (see Hollis's example above and also Chapter 4). This requires a trade of someone's psychological and social wellbeing against absolute physical safety at times (Clarke and Mantle 2016).

Despite new situations and new issues, occupational therapists working with people with dementia and their families and caregivers can consider how occupations and social participation can be enabled. This helps people retain their sense of who they are and what is important to them.

> Susan's driving licence was surrendered after she had an accident in a car park shortly after receiving a dementia diagnosis. Two months later, a local car dealership contacted her home to ask about a new car order that Susan had just placed with them. Susan's daughter cancelled the order. Susan was worried about losing independence and embarrassed at her actions. Susan and her daughter talked this through with the occupational therapist and they problem-solved together how Susan could continue to shop for herself in the small town where she lived. Susan kept a list system of things she needed in a shopping diary, and used sticky labels as visual prompts in the kitchen to check 'use by' dates on fresh ingredients. Her daughter talked through the list with Susan twice a week, and she took this to the local shop where she was known. When Susan found this difficult, she started ordering shopping with her daughter online. This meant Susan could continue to cook at home with ingredients she had chosen.

Some people living with dementia may find they need to transition to a more supported care facility. For many, this transition may follow engagement in community-based activities, or with day support at home or over 24 hours. As with all life in the community, it is important to recognize the role of supporting someone's participation in these new environments, so quality of life and the experience of living with dementia can be best maintained (Brooker 2019). The psychological and social needs of people living with dementia highlighted by Kitwood (1997), and then revisited by Brooker (2019), offer much potential to ensuring that social participation plays an important part in people's lives in that new community-based environment.

Many people with dementia can quickly become institutionalized and deprived of opportunities to fully engage in meaningful occupations, therefore putting them at risk of further physical, psychological and functional deterioration. Unfamiliar environments and routines, lack of stimulation and disengagement from meaningful activities are common features, with particular difficulty being experienced by newly admitted residents who are at most risk of occupational injustices and poor health outcomes.

> Farah had recently moved into a dementia-registered care home after previously living alone at home. She had experienced a rapid deterioration in her independence since the transition into care, and had become anxious, withdrawn and reliant on carers for support with all tasks. Farah was unintentionally given unnecessary assistance by staff members, increasing her sense of task difficulty, and reducing her self-confidence and self-esteem. Consequently, Farah was unable to complete achievable tasks independently. Occupational therapy input involved promoting Farah's abilities, rebuilding her confidence through a graded approach to reintroducing her activities of daily living. Additionally, training care staff became a key process for recognizing and respecting residents' choices, valuing their contribution and promoting social participation. Farah now completes her personal care with minimal prompting. She is involved in arranging the dining hall for mealtimes alongside two other residents she socializes with, and is no longer anxious in her surroundings.

Capacity and consent for people with dementia in community settings

People with dementia have the right to be involved in discussions and to make informed decisions about factors that influence their lives. The ability to make decisions for oneself is termed 'mental capacity'. As dementia progressively affects cognitive functioning, mental capacity is an inherent and prominent issue. People with dementia are more likely than other adults to experience loss of capacity in making decisions about aspects of their daily life. The Mental Capacity Act 2005 is a legal framework to ensure decisions made for individuals without capacity protect their best interests in England and Wales.

'Best interest' decisions about health, care needs, finances and living arrangements can be required as dementia progresses, and help may be sought from family members and caregivers. Throughout their care, the opinions of people with dementia should be encouraged and valued, with efforts made to enhance their understanding by modifying information given or communication methods used. Such decisions should also be in keeping with the wishes and views of the person, their culture and beliefs, and be the least restrictive option possible. Lacking capacity is not definitive for all decisions, so the person with dementia may still be able to make some decisions; they may also lose capacity during a time of illness and regain this once recovered.

Not all decisions incorporate mental capacity, but other important concepts for people with dementia are consent and control. A person living in the community may choose not to engage with services or not accept moving into a care home. They may also refuse help from certain staff and accept it from others. Respecting these choices is important to providing meaningful care and maintaining quality of life.

Sid was recently discharged from hospital with a package of assistance for daily support with personal care. He was keen to get out of hospital and accepted the package. Since returning home, however, he refused access to morning carers, becoming aggressive when they tried to support him. By gathering further information and after discussion with Sid, the occupational therapists established that he did not want to be told what to do in his own home. Sid felt he had lost his sense of control over his life and wanted to maintain his routine of carrying out personal care in the evenings. With flexible support and a collaborative approach, Sid was able to make the informed choice and decision to have support with personal care in the evenings. Sid continues to reside at home and has built a good rapport with the evening care staff.

Conclusion

This chapter has explored the intrinsic link between social participation and health and wellbeing for people with dementia through a community-based lens. It demonstrates the potential of occupational therapy practice to positively address the injustices and in equalities that people with dementia can experience, with examples from community practice. The need for inclusive communities within today's society was discussed, to promote wellbeing and to value and respect all its members.

Reflective questions

1. What steps could widen social participation in a community activity where you live? What advantages would that give to more people?
2. What examples can you find in your community of projects working to combat stigma against people living with dementia? Web search local organizations active in this work. How does this link to the role of occupational therapy discussed in this chapter?
3. Consider your day so far. What environmental barriers can you identify that could stigmatize or exclude a person living with dementia?

References

Alzheimer's Research UK (2020) 'Prevalence.' Dementia Statistics Hub. Accessed on 16/08/2021 at www.dementiastatistics.org/statistics-about-dementia

Alzheimer's Society United Against Dementia (2021) 'Dementia-friendly communities.' London: Alzheimer's Society. Accessed on 03/05/2021 at www.alzheimers.org.uk/get-involved/dementia-friendly-communities

Behr, S.K. and Tebb, S.C. (2016) 'Families and Aging: The Lived Experience'. In K. Barney (ed.) *Occupational Therapy with Aging Adults: Promoting Quality of Life through Collaborative Practice* (Chapter 22). St Louis, MO: Elsevier.

Bekhet, A.K. and Zauszniewski, J.A. (2012) 'Mental health of elders in retirement communities: Is loneliness a key factor?' *Archives of Psychiatric Nursing 26*, 3, 214–224.

Brooker, D. (2019) 'Personhood Maintained.' In T. Kitwood (ed.) *Dementia Reconsidered, Revisited: The Person Still Comes First* (Chapter 4). London: Open University Press, McGraw-Hill Education.

Clarke, C. and Mantle, R. (2016) 'Using risk management to promote person-centred dementia care.' *Nursing Standard 30*, 28, 41–46.

Dawson-Townsend, K. (2019) 'Social participation patterns and their associations with health and well-being for older adults.' *SSM Population Health 8*, 100424. doi:10.1016/j.ssmph.2019.100424. Accessed on 06/09/2021 at www.ncbi.nlm.nih.gov/pmc/articles/PMC6609834

Dementia UK (2020) 'Young onset dementia facts and figures.' London: Dementia UK. Accessed on 14/05/2021 at www.youngdementiauk.org/young-onset-dementia-facts-figures

DH (Department of Health) (2009) *Living Well with Dementia: A National Dementia Strategy*. London: DH. Accessed on 12/08/2021 at https://assets.publishing.service.gov.uk/government/uploads/system/uploads/attachment_data/file/168220/dh_094051.pdf

Fisher, G., Parkinson, S. and Haglund, L. (2017) 'The Environment and Human Occupation.' In R. Taylor (ed.) *Kielhofner's Model of Human Occupation: Theory and Application* (pp.91–122). Philadelphia, PA: Lippincott, Williams & Wilkins.

Iwama, M. (2006) *The Kawa Model: Culturally Relevant Occupational Therapy.* Edinburgh: Churchill Livingstone.

Kinderman, P., Butchard, S., Bruen, A.J., Wall, A., *et al.* (2018) 'A randomised controlled trial to evaluate the impact of a human rights-based approach to dementia care in inpatient ward and care home settings.' *Health Services and Delivery Research 6,* 13. Accessed on 05/11/2021 at https://livrepository.liverpool.ac.uk/3064413/1/3013117.pdf

Kitwood, T. (1997) *Dementia Reconsidered: The Person Comes First.* Buckingham: Open University Press.

Laliberte Rudman, D. (2012) 'Governing through Occupation: Shaping Expectations and Possibilities.' In G.E. Whiteford and C. Hocking (eds) *Occupational Science: Society, Inclusion and Participation* (Chapter 8). Chichester: Wiley-Blackwell.

National Dementia Action Alliance (2021) *The Dementia Statements.* Accessed on 16/08/2021 at www.dementiaaction.org.uk/nationaldementiadeclaration

ONS (Office for National Statistics) (2021) 'Overview of the UK Population: January 2021.' Newport: ONS. Accessed on 12/05/2021 at www.ons.gov.uk/peoplepopulationandcommunity/populationandmigration/populationestimates/articles/overviewoftheukpopulation/january2021

Townsend, E. and Wilcock, A.A. (2004) 'Occupational justice and client centred practice: A dialogue in progress.' *Canadian Journal of Occupational Therapy 71,* 2, 75–87.

Whalley Hammell, K.R. (2013) 'Occupation, wellbeing and culture: Theory and cultural humility.' *Canadian Journal of Occupational Therapy 80,* 4, 224–234

Whiteford, G. (2000) 'Occupational deprivation: Global challenge in the new millennium.' *British Journal of Occupational Therapy 63,* 5, 200–204.

Wilcock, A. and Hocking, C. (2015) *An Occupational Perspective of Health* (3rd edn). Thorofare, NJ: Slack.

CHAPTER 12

Occupation and Rights-Based Practice in Scotland

An Acute Inpatient Setting

Lynsey Robertson and Elizabeth Anne McKay

Learning outcomes

By the end of this chapter, you will have the opportunity to:

- ▸ Understand the complexity of the experience of a person living with dementia in acute inpatient care in general hospitals
- ▸ Identify and explore the enablers and challenges of maintaining human rights in an acute inpatient setting for people living with dementia
- ▸ Consider through the use of a case study how the human rights of people living with dementia can be influenced, and what can be learned from this in an acute occupational therapy inpatient setting
- ▸ Understand capacity and consent in relation to people with dementia having access to meaningful occupations in acute inpatient settings.

Introduction

This chapter explores the experience of people living with dementia receiving care within an acute inpatient hospital setting in Scotland, and the impact that this environment can have on maintaining the human rights of the individual during occupational therapy interventions.

Factors such as the complex physical environment, staff experiences and attitudes are highlighted, along with the effect that these can have on a person living with dementia. These key factors are discussed with reference to a fictional case study based on our experience to consider concepts for occupational therapy practice. We are occupational therapists based in Scotland with practice and personal experience of acute hospital settings and supporting people living with dementia and cognitive change.

Setting the scene

Being an inpatient in an acute hospital can be a worrying time for any older person due to concerns around the reason for admission and the unfamiliar environment of the hospital, all without immediate access to the comfort of friends, family or their own home. For a person living with dementia in particular, being in this environment can be distressing and confusing (NHS Education for Scotland 2016). Acute hospital settings in Scotland, as in other countries, are inherently busy environments, and the demands placed on staff are often high. This can present barriers to being able to provide the level of reassurance required to prevent a person living with dementia experiencing high levels of stress and distress (Digby, Lee and Williams 2016). As Clissett, Porock, Harwood and Gladman (2013) found, priorities within the acute hospital setting often focus on quick turnaround and intervention, which can result in staff practising in a less person-centred manner than settings where turnover is slower.

The following is a fictional case study designed to highlight some of the barriers and opportunities to maintaining the human rights of a person living with dementia receiving care within an acute hospital setting. Mr McDonald's narrative highlights key concepts that are relevant in acute hospital settings.

Mr McDonald is an 83-year-old Scottish gentleman, living with dementia, who was admitted to hospital from home with a hyperactive delirium on a background of a urinary tract infection (UTI) and acute kidney injury. Delirium often occurs when a person has an infection, and can result in increased levels of confusion (Dementia UK 2020). With medical treatment of the underlying infection, delirium can improve within weeks; however, it can also take some months to fully resolve (Dementia UK 2020). Prior to becoming unwell Mr McDonald was living independently at home with his dog Jasper, with no formal support. He has a supportive daughter who lives locally and who visits him most days. He enjoys taking Jasper for walks, attending church and playing golf with his friends. Whilst Mr McDonald does not drive, he is able to access all his leisure activities on foot and walks daily.

On admission, Mr McDonald was extremely distressed and disoriented and made multiple attempts to leave the hospital prior to having received any medical treatment. He was subsequently detained under a short-term detention certificate, as outlined in the Mental Health Care and Treatment Scotland Act 2003. This states that a person can be detained to enable medical or social intervention to protect their wellbeing, health and safety. This was put in place to enable medical staff to administer antibiotics to treat Mr McDonald's UTI, and he was also given a mild sedative.

Human rights, capacity and consent

Maintaining human rights is an important responsibility that all working in health and social care have a duty to ensure is maintained for the people with whom they work (Alzheimer Scotland 2021). This can become more challenging when working with a person living with dementia for a number of reasons. Stavert (2018) highlights the implications of the ongoing use by many of the medical model of disability and manner in which this views 'impairment as a legitimate basis for the denial or restriction of human rights' (Stavert 2018, p.1). The United Nations' Convention on the Rights of Persons with Disabilities (CRPD), (UN 2006) was created with the aim of protecting the human rights and dignity of people with disabilities, and a number of its articles relate directly to practice within the acute hospital setting.

In Mr McDonald's situation, the medical staff used a short-term detention certificate to allow them to maintain his right to freedom and safety (EHRC 2021a). The administration of this must meet strict criteria that ensure the use of detention orders does not undermine the right to liberty (EHRC 2021a).

The use of one-to-one care

> Overnight, Mr McDonald fell. His clinical notes stated this was due to him 'wandering'. He was placed in a side room under one-to-one observation from a clinical support worker.

Adams and Grout (2015) identified that being in hospital can be bewildering for people with dementia or delirium, with staff adopting one-to-one care related to risk management, often with the needs of the service outweighing the needs of the person. Furthermore, one-to-one care is used within acute hospitals when a person is displaying what staff interpret as being dangerous or difficult behaviour. Ward staff may feel that a person living with dementia requires constant care for their own safety. Often the staff member asked to provide the care is based on the needs of the ward rather than the needs of the person receiving the care. For example, a ward manager may allocate a nursing student or clinical support worker to avoid removing registered staff from completing medication administration. As a result of this, the staff member providing constant care may be someone who the person living with dementia has never met, and as such has not had the time to build a therapeutic relationship with (Clissett *et al.* 2013). The staff member may also have limited understanding or experience of dementia.

The intervention being delivered to a person with dementia should always have a therapeutic benefit, be personalized and compassionate. When one-to-one care is provided merely because it is felt to be a necessity, for example as a solution to preventing falls, these values may become difficult to maintain. Putting a person through the undignified experience of being constantly observed by a staff member can be upsetting. It can also breach one of the key principles included within the Charter of Rights for People with Dementia and their Carers in Scotland (Alzheimer Scotland 2009, p.4): 'respect for inherent dignity, individual autonomy including the freedom to make one's own choices, and independence of persons.'

Taking the time to explore possible changes that could be made to the environment and routine of the person with dementia within the ward is supportive of a more ethical and person-centred approach to ensuring an individual's safety. For example, a person may feel more settled and reassured in the company of others, and may cope better in a four-bedded bay as opposed to experiencing isolation in a single room. The availability of shared rooms and single rooms varies between acute settings. Another example would be positioning the person within view of the nurses' station. This way they can be more closely monitored, and nursing staff can intervene if required to ensure their safety, without having to implement constant observation (NHS Education for Scotland 2016). A simple change could have the potential to provide an enhanced, safer experience for both the person admitted and staff members.

The concerns raised by Adams and Grout (2015) regarding the inappropriate use of one-to-one care are reflected in *Dementia Reconsidered, Revisited* (Kitwood 2019), first published by Tom Kitwood in 1997. Here, he discusses the way in which one-to-one care can be a negative and damaging experience for both the person receiving it and the person delivering it. He further explains that delivering care in this manner can create an inappropriate and unnecessary imbalance of power that can result in what he describes as 'projective identification' (2019, p.152). This is a phenomenon during which the caregiver recognizes some of their own childlike and negative personality traits in the person living with dementia, and as such projects these negative feelings onto them. What is subsequently created is a cycle of negative feeling and responses between both parties, which can make an empathetic approach from the professional caregiver very difficult.

In circumstances where one-to-one care is felt to be absolutely necessary and there is an obvious therapeutic benefit, what is happening should be clearly explained to the person living with dementia, as well as their family or caregivers. It is also important to acknowledge that as a result of being detained and moved into a side room, Mr McDonald was being deprived of access to meaningful occupations. According to Whiteford *et al.* (2020), this could be viewed as occupational deprivation as he is being precluded from engaging in occupations due to factors out of his control within the institution. This highlights that time should be taken for rapport to be built between the staff member and the person living with dementia, with a focus on occupational engagement where possible.

Functional assessment

The next morning, the ward occupational therapist and physiotherapist completed a joint initial assessment to gain an understanding of Mr McDonald's functional abilities and needs. Following introductions, time was taken to ask Mr McDonald about his life at home, and he was obviously worried about his dog Jasper. With Mr McDonald's consent the occupational therapist contacted his next of kin (his daughter), and he was reassured that Jasper was being cared for, and he then engaged well with occupational therapy and physiotherapy. This information was handed over to ward staff who were able to consistently reassure Mr McDonald that his dog was in safe hands on the further occasions that he became distressed. Mr McDonald was moved into a bay with three other gentlemen, and nursing staff were able to attend quickly when he became distressed, although his levels of distress were reduced in the company of others.

The occupational therapist continued their assessment for the next seven days, during which time Mr McDonald became more oriented and the medical team felt that his delirium was beginning to resolve, indicating he was medically fit to be discharged home. During occupational therapy input he had stated that he would not be keen on carers supporting him at home. Some professional concerns remained regarding his cognition and the impact that this might have on his safety and participation in occupations after discharge. During a kitchen assessment, Mr McDonald forgot to switch the gas hob off despite prompting, and he continued to have some episodes of disorientation, being unable to recall his address or locate his bed space when he was taken off the ward. He was keen to be discharged home and his daughter wanted to support his wishes. Whilst Mr McDonald was no longer detained, he had an active Adults with Incapacity (Scotland) Certificate – meaning that he was no longer detained, however certain specific medical decisions could be made on his behalf in his best interests if absolutely necessary to protect his wellbeing (legislation.gov.uk 2022).

Having completed a period of functional assessment, the occupational therapist recommended a small package of care to assist Mr McDonald to complete his activities of daily living at home on discharge. In addition to this, there was to be a follow-up from the community occupational therapist for further input and assessment to support him to safely return to engaging in his occupations of importance. A meeting was arranged with Mr McDonald and his daughter. Here, the recommendations were discussed, along with a member of the medical team explaining that his delirium would likely continue to improve, meaning that he may not require carers supporting him at home in the longer term. Taking the time to explain this and that the support would likely be reduced at home allowed Mr McDonald to fully understand the rationale and how this would benefit his safety, and he agreed to a package of care to support him at home.

Occupational therapists working in acute hospital settings in Scotland and other countries often complete a functional assessment. This is to assist the multidisciplinary team's decision-making about whether a person living with dementia can be safely supported to continue living at home. The subsequent outcome of this can be a team decision that a person living with dementia is no longer safe to return to their previous place of residence. The General Medical Council (GMC) in the UK states that, 'Capacity is the ability to make a decision. This ability can vary depending on a patient's condition and how it changes over time, and on the nature of the decision to be made' (GMC 2020, para.76).

A formal capacity assessment and decision must be completed by an appropriately qualified medical professional. If a person living with dementia has been assessed as no longer having capacity to make decisions regarding their home and place of habitation, this decision can be made in what is deemed to be their 'best interests'. Within the acute hospital setting, if a person has been assessed as no longer having capacity and residential care being decided as the safest discharge destination, often the person will be required to remain as an inpatient whilst a suitable placement is found. For those living with dementia, this can limit their access to occupations that are meaningful to them, which Whalley Hammell (2017) argues is a breach of the person's human rights, explaining that a lack of access to meaningful occupation has been found to have a negative impact on wellbeing.

From a human rights perspective, this issue is two-fold. It could be argued that actively stopping a person from returning to their home and the occupations that they engage in within their home environment is a direct violation of their rights (UN 2006). This relates to the right to access a range of environments and to live independently as part of a community (UN 2006), as the person is not being given the opportunity to choose their place of residence or to access community activities. However, occupational therapists have a duty of care to the people who they work with to create safe, appropriate and sustainable discharge plans based on the outcome of a functional assessment. The Royal College of Occupational Therapists' (RCOT) *Professional Standards for Occupational Therapy Practice, Conduct and Ethics* (2021) states that occupational therapists have an obligation to: 'act in the best interests of all those who access the service and those with whom you work, at all times, to ensure their welfare, optimising their health, wellbeing and safety' (RCOT 2021, para.8).

Fundamentally, decisions regarding the most suitable place of discharge for a person living with dementia who has been assessed as no longer having the capacity to make this decision independently must acknowledge and respect the person's beliefs and wishes. Their welfare and the person themselves must also be included in the decision-making process. To achieve this, as with Mr McDonald, family members and/ or caregivers should be included at all stages of the process. Any formal documentation of a person's previously agreed preferences should be investigated, with time taken to discuss this with the person living with dementia through different methods of communication, to ensure all steps are taken to provide an opportunity to explore their wishes and explain the reasoning behind the decisions that are being made. In line with the CRPD (UN 2006), this offers an opportunity for the person's right to respect for family and private life to be maintained.

Article 5 of the European Convention on Human Rights is 'the right to freedom and safety', and the Human Rights Joint Select Committee provides detail and clarity on the circumstances whereby a person can be lawfully detained to maintain their right to freedom and safety:

> Article 5 of the European Convention provides that no one shall be arbitrarily deprived of his or her liberty. There is an exhaustive list of circumstances in which a person can be lawfully deprived of his or her liberty. Article 5(1)(e) provides an exception for the lawful detention of persons of 'unsound mind', subject to certain minimum conditions. (UK Parliament 2018, para.17)

Therefore, to maintain the human rights of a person living with dementia when they have been assessed as not having capacity whilst remaining as an inpatient for further assessment to determine the most appropriate discharge plan, it is essential that all possible avenues are explored to identify the least restrictive option. The decision must be made with the inclusion of the entire multidisciplinary team, including a psychiatrist, the person with dementia and members of their family. Regardless of the stage of progression of the person living with dementia, it is important that the reasoning behind the recommendations is clearly explained to them and repeated as often as required. A person living with dementia can find the experience of not being allowed to leave the hospital extremely distressing, and constant reassurance and explanation should be provided to them.

Protecting human rights

Taking steps via clinical input and assessment to protect a person's right to safety could, in turn, present a challenge to maintaining human rights when there may be a heightened perception of risk from the multidisciplinary team and an over-application of the principle of aiming to protect the person's safety. It is imperative that occupational therapists ensure that a balance remains between ensuring a person's safety is protected and protecting their liberty, by identifying and proceeding with the least restrictive option at all times. This includes advocating for reduced occupational deprivation and access to meaningful occupations.

Discharge planning

Both Mr McDonald and his daughter had been clear that Mr McDonald's priority was to return home at the earliest opportunity. Using the available community services, including accessing a package of care and community occupational therapy input, allowed the occupational therapist to create a safe discharge plan to support discharge home.

The action of taking time to discuss what was important to Mr McDonald, including his daughter in the assessment process, and ensuring he could be discharged home as safely and swiftly as possible were all steps that worked towards protecting his 'right to respect for private and family life, home and correspondence' (EHRC 2021b).

The input from the occupational therapist in Mr McDonald's case illustrates how attention to the simple aspects of a person's life at home and developing a therapeutic relationship can help to maintain their rights. Thinking back to the idea of 'projective identification' (Kitwood 2019) discussed earlier, this could present a potential risk to the development of a therapeutic relationship, and as such, could be a barrier to respecting and maintaining the rights of the person.

Providing a dementia-friendly inpatient acute service

A range of initiatives is available to support people living with dementia and their caregivers when a person is admitted into an acute hospital setting. One such example relates to interpreting pain. A person living with dementia can often experience difficulties interpreting and communicating feelings of pain, which can, in turn, increase levels of stress and distress. The OUCH! (Observe, Understand, Communicate and Help) campaign was launched by the Royal Wolverhampton NHS Trust (2018) with the aim of increasing awareness amongst clinical staff of understanding the experience of pain in dementia. This is an encouraging example of positive steps being taken to create a workforce of clinical staff who have the required skills and knowledge to provide effective inpatient care to people living with dementia. The Dementia Action Alliance (DAA) published the *Dementia-Friendly Hospital Charter* (2018), which encompasses helpful self-assessment sections that can be used by hospital staff to identify areas that can be improved.

Despite the initiatives in place to support dementia-friendly environments and practice, there is still a long way to go towards the creation of a truly dementia-friendly workforce within acute hospitals. The disappointing reality is that ongoing challenges in relation to staffing within hospitals mean that often the overall patient experience of a person with dementia is compromised.

So often time pressures, high staff turnover and lack of awareness are what prevent ward-based staff from being able to really get to know a person living with dementia within the inpatient hospital setting (Digby *et al.* 2016). Occupational therapists and students are in a prime position to spend time with people to find strategies to help communication and identify what is important to them, and to then set appropriate, meaningful goals and discharge plans. From experience, the occupational therapy team is frequently in contact with the family and caregivers of a person living with dementia, which provides an opportunity to build a rapport with the people closest to the person, allowing additional opportunities to find out what is important to the person to help guide any interventions.

Conclusion

Within the acute inpatient care setting there are numerous opportunities and barriers to maintaining the human rights of a person living with dementia. Whilst this chapter has explored some of these, it is a multifaceted area. As occupational therapists, we all have a responsibility to ensure the human rights of those under our care are maintained and respected during all our input. For people living with dementia, ensuring that their voice is always heard is an important step that we must take to maintain their rights. This can be achieved through taking time to find the most appropriate method of communication for the person, careful observation, and including family members and caregivers throughout their inpatient journey and discharge planning.

Reflective questions

1. What are your thoughts on the use of the term 'wandering' within the case study, and what might be a better, more person-centred way to describe Mr McDonald's overnight activity, and why?
2. In what way did Mr McDonald's inpatient experience change once staff became aware of his worries about his dog Jasper?
3. As an occupational therapist, what steps will you take to ensure that all interventions consider, promote and respect the human rights of the people with whom you work?

References

Adams, S. and Grout, G. (2015) 'When should I use one-to-one nursing for a patient with dementia or delirium?' Nursing Older People, 26 November. Accessed on 26/11/2021 at https://rcni.com/nursing-older-people/evidence-and-practice/practice-question/when-should-i-use-one-one-one-nursing

Alzheimer Scotland (2009) *Charter of Rights for People with Dementia and their Carers in Scotland*. Accessed on 17/05/2022 at www.alzscot.org/sites/default/files/images/0000/2678/Charter_of_Rights.pdf

Alzheimer Scotland (2021) 'Rights based approach to dementia.' Edinburgh: Alzheimer Scotland. Accessed on 26/11/2021 at www.alzscot.org/our-work/campaigning-for-change/rights-based-approach-to-dementia

Clissett, P., Porock, D., Harwood, R.H. and Gladman, J.R.F. (2013) 'The challenges of achieving person-centred care in acute hospitals: A qualitative study of people with dementia and their families.' *International Journal of Nursing Studies 50*, 11, 1495–1503.

DAA (Dementia Action Alliance) (2018) *Dementia-Friendly Hospital Charter, Revised 2018*. Accessed on 26/11/21 at www.dementiaaction.org.uk/assets/0003/9960/DEMENTIA-FRIENDLY_HOSPITAL_CHARTER_2018_FINAL.pdf

Dementia UK (2020) 'Delirium (sudden confusion).' Accessed on 26/11/2021 at https://www.dementiauk.org/get-support/understanding-changes-in-behaviour/delirium

Digby, R., Lee, S. and Williams, A. (2016) 'The experience of people with dementia and nurses in hospital: An integrative review.' *Journal of Clinical Nursing 26*, 9–10, 1152–1171.

EHRC (Equality and Human Rights Commission) (2021a) 'Article 5: Right to liberty and security.' Accessed on 26/11/2021 at www.equalityhumanrights.com/en/human-rights-act/article-5-right-liberty-and-security

EHRC (2021b) 'Article 8: Respect for your private and family life.' Accessed on 26/11/2021 at www.equalityhumanrights.com/en/human-rights-act/article-8-respect-your-private-and-family-life

GMC (General Medical Council) (2020) 'Circumstances that affect the decision-making process continued.' Manchester: GMC. Accessed on 26/11/2021 at www.gmc-uk.org/ethical-guidance/ethical-guidance-for-doctors/decision-making-and-consent/circumstances-that-affect-the-decision-making-process-continued-2

Kitwood, T. (1997) *Dementia Reconsidered: The Person Comes First*. Buckingham: Open University Press.

Kitwood, T. (2019) *Dementia Reconsidered, Revisited: The Person Still Comes First* (edited by D. Brooker). London: Open University Press, McGraw Hill Education.

Legislation.gov.uk (2022) 'Adults with Incapacity (Scotland) Act 2000.' Accessed on 02/06/2022 at https://www.legislation.gov.uk/asp/2000/4/contents

Mental Health (Care and Treatment) (Scotland) Act (2003). Accessed on 26/11/2021 at www.legislation.gov.uk/asp/2003/13/contents

NHS Education for Scotland (2016) *Supporting People with Dementia in Acute Care: Learning Resource*. Edinburgh: NHS Education for Scotland. Accessed on 26/11/2021 at www.knowledge.scot.nhs.uk/media/11866144/supporting%20people%20with%20dementia%20in%20acute%20care%20final%202016%20web.pdf

RCOT (Royal College of Occupational Therapists) (2021) *RCOT Professional Standards for Occupational Therapy Practice, Conduct and Ethics*. London: RCOT. Accessed on 25/04/2022 at www.rcot.co.uk/publications/professional-standards-occupational-therapy-practice-conduct-and-ethics

Royal Wolverhampton NHS Trust (2018) 'OUCH! – Understanding pain in dementia care.' Press release, 21 May. Accessed on 26/11/2021 at www.royalwolverhampton.nhs.uk/media/press-release-archive/press-releases-2018/may-2018/ouch-understanding-pain-in-dementia-care

Stavert, J. (2018) 'Paradigm shift or paradigm paralysis? National Mental Health and Capacity Law implementing the CRPD in Scotland.' *Laws 7*, 3, 1–15.

UK Parliament (2018) 'The Right to Freedom and Safety: Reform of the Deprivation of Liberty Safeguards, 2 Legal Framework, Article 5 European Convention on Human Rights.' Accessed on 26/11/2021 at https://publications.parliament.uk/pa/jt201719/jtselect/jtrights/890/89005.htm

UN (United Nations) (2006) 'Convention on the Rights of Persons with Disabilities (CRPD).' Accessed on 26/11/2021 at www.un.org/development/desa/disabilities/convention-on-the-rights-of-persons-with-disabilities.html

Whalley Hammell, K.R. (2017) 'Opportunities for well-being: The right to occupational engagement.' *Canadian Journal of Occupational Therapy 84*, 4–5, 209–222.

Whiteford, G., Jones, K., Weekes, G., Ndlovu, N., *et al.* (2020) 'Combatting occupational deprivation and advancing occupational justice in institutional settings: Using a practice-based enquiry approach for service transformation.' *British Journal of Occupational Therapy 83*, 1, 52–61.

CHAPTER 13

The Pool Activity Level (PAL) Instrument

An Occupational Focus for Engagement, Function and Wellbeing

Jackie Pool, Liz Copley and Sophia Dickinson

Learning outcomes

By the end of this chapter, you will have the opportunity to:

▶ Gain an understanding of the historical, theoretical and research perspectives of the development of the PAL Instrument to improve your confidence in its use
▶ Review real-life examples of the application of the PAL Instrument in a variety of clinical settings to plan for implementation in your own service
▶ Critique the strengths and limitations of the PAL Instrument to understand how and when to use it in your own practice.

How the Pool Activity Level (PAL) Instrument came to be

The history of how and why I, Jackie Pool, developed the Pool Activity Level (PAL) Instrument might be of interest to occupational therapists because it provides some insights into the role of the profession in developing instruments to meet the clinical needs of the people we work with, rather than trying to work with what is available to us even though it might not be fit for the purpose. In the early 1990s, I supported an occupational therapist to develop activity provision in a group of local authority care homes. The occupational therapist used the Allen Cognitive Levels Screen (ACLS) and understanding of the Cognitive Disabilities Model (CDM) (Allen, Earhart and Blue 1992) to assess each resident's cognitive function, and then used clinical reasoning skills to draw inferences from the assessment outcome that would shape the activity plan for the individual.

At the same time, I was also working alongside the University of Bradford Dementia Group (now the Centre for Applied Dementia Studies), to deliver what was then ground-breaking training on person-centred approaches in dementia. The late Professor Tom Kitwood, head of the group, with whom I worked closely delivering courses and developing materials, requested that I contribute a text on the enablement of individuals to perform activities of daily living (ADL).

Our discussions on that text plus my work with the local authority came together in a serendipitous moment that resulted in the first concept of the PAL Instrument as a tool for supporting caregivers (formal and informal), a self-interpreting tool that caregivers and activity providers could use to enable people living with dementia to engage in meaningful occupation, and therefore to optimize their function and wellbeing. My idea was to draw on the model underpinning Allen's assessment to develop an instrument that would identify the cognitive functional level by observation of everyday ADL, and crucially that would self-interpret to produce a guide for those supporting the individual at their level of ability.

Theoretical perspective

It will be no surprise, therefore, that the main influencers on the development of the PAL Instrument are the late Claudia Kay Allen's CDM (Allen *et al.* 1992) and Tom Kitwood's person-centred model of dementia (Kitwood 1997).

The CDM had its beginnings at the Eastern Pennsylvania Psychiatric Institute in the late 1960s when Claudia Kay Allen, an occupational therapist, and her colleagues first observed patterns of performance difficulties in adult patients with mental disorders. Allen (1985) began a systematic collection of observations focusing on sensorimotor actions that influence routine task behaviour that could be observed and assessed. The construct of functional cognition has since become a useful term for describing the focus of concern of the CDM (McCraith, Austin and Earhart 2011). The model defines cognitive functioning in the way that it affects the person's engagement in occupation and with others (Pool 2011).

Allen proposed six cognitive levels, ranging from coma (0.8) to normal (6.0). Each level has three components: attention, motor and verbal performance. There is a battery of assessment instruments to determine the specific level of ability, and the ACLS (Allen *et al.* 2007) is commonly used in the UK. This is a lacing activity that assesses problem-solving and new learning by the performance of three different stitches, from simple to complex. It is used as a predictor of occupational performance given the level of cognitive functional ability, and the occupational therapist translates these findings into a treatment programme.

Functional cognition encompasses the complex and dynamic interactions between an individual's cognitive abilities and the activity context that produces observable performance. The PAL Instrument contains a checklist that identifies a person's overall cognitive functional level from Allen's levels, from 0.8 to 5.8, by describing the person's ability to engage in nine functional domains. As with Allen's model, descriptions of the PAL Instrument domains are based on cognitive development theory (Piaget 1952; Vygotsky 1978), with each domain providing four descriptions that are aligned to the executive function stages of these theorists: planned, exploratory, sensory and reflex (see Table 13.1).

Table 13.1. PAL Instrument levels description with relationship to Allen's Cognitive Levels Screen

PAL Instrument levels	Reflex	Sensory	Exploratory	Planned
ACLS	0.8–1.8	2.0–3.4	3.5–4.8	5.0–5.8
Likely abilities	Can make reflex responses to direct sensory stimulation	Is likely to be responding to bodily sensations	Can carry out very familiar activities in familiar surroundings	Can explore different ways of carrying out an activity

PAL Instrument levels	Reflex	Sensory	Exploratory	Planned
ACLS	0.8–1.8	2.0–3.4	3.5–4.8	5.0–5.8
Likely limitations	May not be aware of the surrounding environment or even their own body	May not have any conscious plan to carry out a movement to achieve a particular end result	May not have an end result in mind when starting activities	May not be able to solve problems that arise
Caregiver's role	To enable the person to be more aware of themselves	To enable the person to experience the effect of the activity on their senses	To enable the person to experience the sensation of doing the activity rather than focusing on the end result	To enable the person to take control of the activity and to master the steps involved

After completion of the checklist, users identify the level of the person's cognitive functional ability by the majority of levels selected across the nine domains. They can then select from one of the four PAL profiles, each describing how to present an activity to the person at their level of ability, to optimize occupational performance, social engagement and wellbeing.

Kitwood (1997) advocated the importance of personhood in meaningful interaction and engagement, and led the way for a global understanding of dementia as a group of symptoms not only resulting from neurological impairment but also impacted on by the individual's unique perspective of their personality, biography, physical and mental health and their social-psychological experience. The PAL Instrument includes a personal history profile so that the unique biography of the individual can be understood in the context of planning meaningful activity at the appropriate level of the person.

In 2020, Quality Compliance Systems (QCS) acquired the PAL Instrument. Following registration there is now a free download of the

PAL Instrument (QCS 2020), with an expansion of the PAL profile into a more comprehensive PAL guide that details how to support the person in five ADL: bathing, showering and washing; getting dressed; dining; engaging with others; and engaging in leisure activities. The guide also includes space to record the person's preferences and routines for each of these activities and, in addition, provides some tips for creating an enabling task environment. These further developments of the PAL Instrument ensure that a truly person-centred framework is delivered in practice.

Reliability and validity of the PAL Instrument for people with dementia

The first version of the PAL Instrument contained the checklist and profiles. They were trialled with a group of UK care homes as well as by occupational therapy colleagues in an older people's mental health inpatient and community-based service. Feedback helped to shape it, and it was first published in 1999.

Wenborn et al. (2008) studied the reliability and validity of the PAL checklist when used with older people with dementia with two phases to the study. Phase One investigated the content validity, assessing the intended PAL checklist concept of the individual's cognitive ability to engage in activity. This used a postal questionnaire that was sent out to 122 occupational therapists and activity providers from the College of Occupational Therapists (COT) Specialist Section for Older People, Dementia Forum, and from the National Activity Providers Association. The questionnaire response rate was 83 per cent (102/122). Most respondents felt no important items were missing. Seven of the nine activities were ranked as 'very important' or 'essential' by at least 77 per cent of the sample, indicating very good content validity.

Validity and reliability were measured in a sample of 60 older people with dementia. Correlation with measures of cognition, severity of dementia and activity performance demonstrated strong concurrent validity. Inter-item correlation indicated strong construct validity. Cronbach's alpha coefficient measured internal consistency as excellent (0.95). All items achieved acceptable test-retest reliability, and the majority demonstrated acceptable inter-rater reliability. Wenborn et al. (2008) concluded that the PAL Instrument checklist demonstrates adequate validity and reliability when used with older people with dementia, and appears a useful instrument for a variety of care settings.

Availability and forms of the PAL Instrument

The PAL Instrument began to be increasingly used across different care settings, providing an evidence base for health and social care practice. Following further feedback from occupational therapists on their use of the PAL Instrument, the second edition was published in 2002 and included a life history profile to support the person-centred approach to using it. Further editions were published in 2008 and 2012, with additional case study examples and more information on the use of sensory environments. Because of the standardization of the PAL Instrument checklist, it has also been used as an assessment instrument within research studies into the impact of health and social care delivery.

The entire PAL Instrument book was translated into Japanese and made culturally relevant in 2012, and into Lithuanian in 2019, by Jessica Kingsley Publishers. In addition, the PAL Instrument has been translated into Danish, German and Spanish, and is used by occupational therapists in those countries as well as in many other English-speaking countries, including Australia and the USA.

Use of the PAL Instrument in occupational therapy clinical practice

The PAL Instrument was first developed to support those without the necessary experience or understanding of how to engage people with dementia in meaningful activity, which is a core skill of occupational therapists. It is being used successfully by family members, caregivers and support workers and activity providers in a range of hospital, residential, community and clinical settings. An occupational therapist is well placed to supervise the completion of the PAL Instrument checklist and to share advice using the PAL Instrument guide or profile.

It is also a helpful standardized instrument for occupational therapists in inpatient, reablement and community settings to plan rehabilitation and therapeutic interventions with the aim of developing higher functional skills, using the initial checklist outcome as a baseline, and then repeating it after a series of interventions to evaluate the impact of the treatment.

Occupational therapists who support residential care homes and domiciliary care providers can also use the PAL Instrument to enable a consistent approach in supporting personal care activities. The PAL Instrument also facilitates meaningful living for people with dementia with an informed approach to the provision of planned or spontaneous leisure activities.

In an NHS Trust in England, the PAL Instrument is used across inpatient wards, community teams and in a specialist pathway for individuals living with dementia in care homes who express distress through their behaviour. The PAL Instrument is viewed, in this service, as having a key role in assessments, which also includes an observation phase to complete two weeks of behaviour record charts, and a distressed behaviour scale. The checklist is usually completed by support staff in partnership with care home staff and family, including the life history and an interest checklist. Support staff also have initial discussions with care home staff about individualized care in line with the relevant PAL Instrument guide, and provide advice and some short-term input around individualized therapy programmes and activities. The team occupational therapist provides supervision to support staff throughout this as well as offering direct observed assessment and support with developing the guide in depth with the care team.

The independent occupational therapy practitioner can also find use of the PAL Instrument supportive to their service, evidencing their practice and increasing confidence when often in a lone-working situation, without the support of a manager or a peer.

To maintain confidentiality, pseudonyms are used in the following case studies to represent aspects of work known to us, although specific details are excluded.

CASE STUDY 1: RE-ENGAGING IN MEANINGFUL ACTIVITY

Harry, aged 79, had a diagnosis of mixed dementia, with a history of mild cerebral vascular accidents and some physical changes and mild mobility problems. He was referred to the Community Mental Health

Team (CMHT) as his wife, Anne, said she was unable to cope much longer. She said that Harry was argumentative and just sat 'doing nothing', no longer carrying out previous activities. Anne described how Harry could be independent with basic self-care, but not to his previous standards, and she had to remind him to have a wash and complete tasks. Often when asked to do things he would just say he had already completed the task, even though he had not.

Harry used to be a member of his local Bowling Club, and would go out to meetings regularly, but had stopped attending because he could not remember the names of the other members. He had also been a keen gardener, growing vegetables, but would not now go into the garden unless persuaded.

Anne spoke of feeling guilty about losing her temper, but believed that Harry could do more and that he was at times deliberately being difficult. They were both distressed by the situation and describe a happy marriage and busy family life prior to Harry's dementia diagnosis. The couple also had two adult sons, both living close by with their own families.

The occupational therapy assessment included the PAL Instrument checklist (Pool 2012), Harry's life story and an interest checklist.

The life story information revealed that Harry had worked as a painter and decorator until his retirement. He described himself as a 'quiet family man' who liked to learn new things, enjoyed reading, crosswords and sport. He also had played amateur league football for a local team and remained involved with them.

Harry's sons and grandchildren used to be 'always in and out' of their house, and used to go together to football training and matches, although all this had now stopped. Anne said Harry did not seem bothered anymore and the grandchildren had stopped calling. Harry's sons said they would like to help but felt upset and were unsure how to help.

Observation of the home environment revealed that the bathroom and bedroom were cluttered and the wardrobes were overfull with clothing. Piles of newspapers and correspondence were on all the surfaces, making it difficult to find things.

Completion of the PAL Instrument checklist revealed that Harry was functioning at an exploratory level in seven of the domains and at a planned level in the two domains of bathing and washing and looking at a newspaper or magazine. Therefore, Harry's overall PAL Instrument level was at an exploratory level.

Completing the PAL Instrument exploratory level guide with Harry and his family meant it was highly personalized. It was a great way to educate the family about his needs and abilities and the practical ways they could support him, particularly around setting up and initiating tasks. The family was supported to focus on positive actions to remove clutter and items causing barriers, particularly in the bathroom and bedroom. Once this was done, Harry's clothing and other items were more simply organized, so it was easier for him to see things, to use visual cues and procedural routines and skills to initiate and sequence tasks.

Using the PAL Instrument guide also helped in terms of building compassion and enabling Harry's family to adapt and adjust their expectations. It was used as the basis for specific goals around a daily/weekly routine, including simple crosswords and garden tasks.

Harry's sons thought of ways their dad could resume a role in football, and they started going to the club again. Using the PAL Instrument exploratory guide, this included the need to remind him of day/time, steps and set-up so he was helped to get ready. This approach changed the focus from whether or not he wanted to or 'was bothered', and set a different narrative based on his abilities – that he still could have a meaningful role and that they wanted to be with him. It really helped everyone recognize and support tasks he could be involved in, matched to his abilities and in line with the exploratory level guide. Harry took on the role of folding raffle tickets for the half-time draw, time-keeping on the sideline, blowing the whistle when asked in between coaching activities and giving out kit alongside other volunteers.

Good outcomes were reported from Harry's family as arguments and frustrations had reduced and they had adjusted to the changes well. The sons were in contact later, saying that they still went with Harry to football even when he could do less, that they had accepted this, and whilst he mainly sat quietly watching, he would also take charge of the bag for team drinks. They were glad he was there and could be part of family life.

CASE STUDY 2: RE-ESTABLISHING SELF-CONFIDENCE AND SELF-ESTEEM

George, 85, fell frequently and required physical assistance to lift him up from the floor. He had broken his clavicle after a fall and his wife had injured her back trying to help him up from the floor. George had a diagnosis of vascular dementia, which was in the early to moderate stages. He had attended two falls clinics and could mobilize 30 metres with a walking frame, although he sometimes struggled with his coordination and balance. George had some awareness of his diagnosis and said he sometimes felt confused and forgetful. He spent most of the time watching television or reading the newspaper. George's wife Sarah had adopted the caregiver role and did most things for him. George said that he felt frustrated and wished that he could do more to help.

George was a retired bank manager who loved reading and was knowledgeable on many subjects, including history, politics and all things engineering. He also enjoyed watching football on the television and playing it in the garden with his two grandchildren.

The couple lived in a ground-floor flat with a slight ramp at the front access, no internal steps and a level access shower with a wall-fixed shower seat. George could recall that he had fallen frequently in the shower room, and reported that the falls took place in the evening when he was negotiating the corners in the hallway.

Practical solutions to reduce the risk of further falls were implemented, including highlighting the corners with a contrasting tape or brightly coloured paint plus increased lighting in the hallway. Further environmental modifications included assistive technology items, such as a bed and chair sensor and shower chair.

George also needed to engage in meaningful and therapeutically beneficial activities that would improve his strength, stamina, balance and coordination. This would not only address the underlying cause of his falls but would also support his role identity by encouraging a balanced relationship with his wife. The PAL Instrument was used as it is user-friendly and informative, easy to interpret, apply and share with George's family.

The book-based version of the PAL Instrument checklist (Pool 2012) was completed with George and Sarah, and identified that he was at the planned level in five domains and at an exploratory level in four (getting dressed, contact with others, group work skills and use of objects). Therefore, his overall PAL Instrument level was planned. The PAL Instrument activity profile was shared with Sarah, who could see George's likely abilities and limitations, and that part of the caregiver's role was to encourage involvement and to enable him to take more control of activities.

Sarah seemed pleased to have a clear direction and assisted by completing a leisure interest checklist and a personal history profile. This helped gain a better picture of the significant events and experiences in George's life and enhanced the therapeutic relationship. With this information, a therapeutically meaningful activity was developed with George and Sarah. This was aimed at promoting George's long-term memory, enhancing his wellbeing and promoting physical exercise to increase his strength, balance and endurance.

As George missed playing football with his grandson and granddaughter, he was motivated to engage in football-related therapy with the aim of improving his mobility and confidence. They commenced the activity by playing the *Match of the Day* theme tune and looking at pictures of George's grandchildren to facilitate conversation. George's walking frame was positioned as the goal two metres in front of George and Sarah whilst they were seated. The game involved a competition between George and Sarah to see who could score the most goals. There was a wonderful atmosphere, with lots of praise and clapping when a goal was scored. Sarah laughed and George expressed his delight at having won the game. As described in the PAL Instrument activity profile for the planned level of ability, introducing competitiveness was indeed highly effective in creating fun and raising mood and feelings of wellbeing.

The PAL Instrument was helpful in guiding the occupational therapy intervention. George's goals were achieved, and he demonstrated a sense of achievement. At the start of each session George was asked to rate his feelings and again after each session, and a consistent increase was observed after three sessions. George's non-verbal communication and use of language and tone of voice was also assessed for his sense of enjoyment and wellbeing.

The PAL Instrument empowered George's family, who were able to apply it with additional activities including discussing daily newspaper headlines and completing jigsaw puzzles to promote his ability to problem-solve and sequence tasks, and to be oriented in time by discussing current affairs.

Strengths of the PAL Instrument:

- Reliability and validity
- Quick to complete
- Supports purposeful practice in meaningful activities
- Supports family caregivers
- Simple, quick and easy to complete
- Helps with education around dementia
- Provides practical and reliable means of addressing changing needs and abilities.

Limitations of the PAL Instrument:

- Not a diagnostic measure
- Not suitable for those with physical impairments that are impacting on function
- The person must sometimes be observed as it is a measure of what they can do and not what they are doing
- Best completed as a group discussion as the person with dementia might not show their level of ability to one person or in one observed situation.

Conclusion

It is our view that the strength of the PAL Instrument is its reliability and validity and that it is not only simple to complete, but that it also provides practical and reliable means of addressing changing needs and abilities – supporting purposeful and meaningful engagement. Whilst it is not a tool that should be used when it is a physical impairment that is impacting on functional ability, it is certainly useful for education and delivery of clinical services to enable the potential of those who are living with dementia.

Reflective questions

1. Can you think of how you would apply the PAL Instrument in a group setting?
2. In what ways could you apply the PAL Instrument to accommodate sensory deficits such as visual or auditory impairments?
3. What would you need to consider to introduce the use of the PAL Instrument into a new setting, and how would you support other multidisciplinary team colleagues to use it competently?

References

Allen, C.K. (1985). *Occupational Therapy for Psychiatric Diseases: Measurement and Management of Cognitive Disabilities.* Boston, MA; Little, Brown, & Company. [No longer in print.]

Allen, C.K., Earhart, C.A. and Blue, T. (1992) *Occupational Therapy Treatment Goals for the Physically and Cognitively Disabled.* Rockville, MD: The American Occupational Therapy Association.

Allen, C.K., Austin, S., David, S., Earhart, C., McCraith, D. and Riska-Williams, L. (2007) *Manual for the Allen Cognitive Level Screen (ACLS-5) and Large Allen Cognitive Level Screen (LACLS-5).* Camarillo, CA: ACLS and LACLS Committee.

Kitwood, T. (1997) *Dementia Reconsidered: The Person Comes First.* Buckingham: Open University Press.

McCraith, D.B., Austin, S.L. and Earhart, C.A. (2011) 'The Cognitive Disabilities Model in 2011'. In N. Katz (ed.) *Cognition, Occupation, and Participation across the Life Span: Neuroscience, Neurorehabilitation, and Models of Intervention in Occupational Therapy* (3rd edn). White Plains, MD: American Occupational Therapy Association.

Piaget, J. (1952) *The Origins of Intelligence in Children.* New York: International Universities Press.

Pool, J. (2011) 'The Functional Information-Processing Model.' In E. Duncan (ed.) *Foundations for Practice in Occupational Therapy* (4th edn, pp.105–115). Edinburgh: Elsevier.

Pool, J. (2012 [1999]) *The Pool Activity Level (PAL) Instrument for Occupational Profiling.* London: Jessica Kingsley Publishers.

QCS (Quality Compliance Systems) (2020) 'Digital Pool Activity Level (PAL) Instrument.' Accessed on 08/12/2021 at www.qcs.co.uk/digital-pool-activity-level-pal-instrument

Vygotsky, L.S. (1978) *The Development of Higher Psychological Processes.* Boston, MA: Harvard University Press.

Wenborn, J., Challis, D., Pool, J., Burgess, J., Elliott, N. and Orrell, M. (2008) 'Assessing the validity and reliability of the Pool Activity Level (PAL) checklist for use with older people with dementia.' *Aging & Mental Health 12,* 2, 202–211.

CHAPTER 14

Occupational Therapy Home Based Memory Rehabilitation (OTHBMR)

An Improvement Project in Practice

Alison McKean, Mary McGrath and Gill Gowran

Learning outcomes
By the end of this chapter, you will have the opportunity to:

▸ Understand the purpose, design and delivery of Occupational Therapy Home Based Memory Rehabilitation (OTHBMR) as an individualized, rehabilitative, post-diagnostic intervention for people living with dementia and their caregivers
▸ Explore the theory and principles underpinning OTHBMR, including its focus on occupation, routine and structure
▸ Consider the importance of ongoing evaluation connected to delivery of OTHBMR across occupational therapy services
▸ Reflect on how the OTHBMR strategies are used by a person living with dementia.

Introduction

The World Health Organization (WHO) (2020) defines rehabilitation as a set of interventions designed to optimize functioning and reduce disability in individuals with health conditions in interaction with their environment. Specifically, the WHO (2017) *Global Action Plan on the Public Health Response to Dementia* promotes community-based rehabilitation as an effective strategy that can enable and support people living with dementia to preserve their autonomy and rights. This is supported by an emerging evidence base highlighting the need for people living with dementia to access rehabilitation, with published work by Marshall (2005), literature reviews by Ravn, Petersen and Thuesen (2019) and Jogie *et al.* (2021), and a textbook edited by Low and Laver (2021) that includes a range of evidence-based interventions. This includes, for example, occupational therapy, exercise programmes, psychological therapy and working with families to optimize independence. However, evidence also indicates that access to rehabilitation programmes that aim to respond to the symptoms of dementia are often still not routinely available (Cations *et al.* 2020).

Consequently, this chapter will share one example of an individualized, tailored and early rehabilitation intervention for people living with dementia, known as Occupational Therapy Home Based Memory Rehabilitation (OTHBMR). This rehabilitation approach aims to enhance and maintain for longer a person's occupational performance, and is now being routinely offered as a post-diagnostic intervention across Northern Ireland and Scotland.

The chapter begins by describing in brief the underpinning theory informing OTHBMR, highlighting what the occupational therapy intervention is, and how it is being evaluated as part of everyday occupational therapy practice. Finally, a case study highlighting the use of OTHBMR strategies adopted by a person living with dementia is presented.

Underpinning theory informing OTHBMR

OTHBMR was developed by one of the authors (Mary) as part of her early research, the aim of which was to respond to an identified gap in post-diagnostic occupational therapy service provision for people living with dementia and their caregivers. The intention of the research was to design and evaluate a rehabilitation intervention that could support and enable people living with dementia to compensate for memory difficulties, and to maintain their independence and safety at home for as long as possible (McGrath 2013; McGrath and Passmore 2009). The review of literature in advance of the creation of OTHBMR identified three key elements of practice, considered below.

Memory rehabilitation

Early work by Wilson and Hughes (1997) suggests memory rehabilitation constitutes one part of cognitive rehabilitation. Cognitive rehabilitation is recognized and defined by the National Institute for Health and Care Excellence (NICE) (2018, p.21) as 'improving or maintaining functioning in everyday life, building on the person's strengths, and finding ways to compensate for impairments, and supporting independence.' It is a collaborative process involving people with dementia setting personal goals that aim to reduce the impact of functional difficulties experienced in everyday life (Clare 2017; Clare *et al.* 2019). The key concept of memory rehabilitation is to enable people with memory difficulties to compensate for any deficits. The compensatory approach constitutes two main areas: the use of external memory aids, or an aide memoir, and environmental adaptation to support these strategies. This influenced the development of OTHBMR by creating and integrating the use of memory aids (outlined below), to prompt and support memory retrieval. In dementia, of course, memory function does not deteriorate in isolation, and can be affected by deficits in other areas of cognition, including attention.

Pay attention to attention

Attention is a cornerstone for all cognitive functions including memory (Maskill and Tempest 2017). The more complex the cognitive function, the higher the level of attention required. Indeed, the relationship between attention and memory can be compared to the interaction of the bridge (memory) and the engine room (attention) on a ship. For the safe and successful operation of the ship, both elements must be functioning well and working in harmony.

Early in dementia, attention begins to falter, and this may initially affect complex attention. Sohlberg and Mateer (2001), who have considered the important contribution of cognitive rehabilitation more widely, suggest an example of this is divided attention that can support multitasking. As attention deteriorates further, the ability to sustain attention and complete a task can falter (Maskill and Tempest 2017). It has been observed in practice that constant failure to complete tasks has a detrimental effect on the self-confidence of the person with dementia. Distractors such as pain, depression, anxiety, bereavement, trauma and the effects of medication can also affect the quality of attention.

Practice and rehearsal are therefore core components of OTHBMR to help reduce reliance on attention and to rebuild confidence.

Compensation for attention deficits

Compensation for attention deficits includes optimizing hearing and vision along with practical advice for the person to avoid multitasking, and where the person is encouraged to do one thing at a time. It can be difficult for people living with dementia to divide their attention, so focus on one thing at a time to promote, as far as possible, success. Caregiver education is integral, encouraging them to enable the person with dementia to maintain and sustain attention and complete a task by not interrupting, for example waiting until the person has finished preparing a hot drink before conversing about plans later that day. Adapting the environment to reduce distractions and minimize background noise such as the television whilst also ensuring good lighting, adequate heating and ventilation ensures that the person is as comfortable as possible, which helps them to focus and concentrate on an occupation.

In summary, the three approaches described above were embedded into OTHBMR to develop an intervention that can help to create structure and repetition to encourage new learned behaviours in the early stages of dementia, and habits and routines that are identified, highlighted and emphasized so they are more likely to be remembered and relied on as memory difficulties progress.

Delivering OTHBMR

The OTHBMR intervention has been adopted in health and social care trusts in Northern Ireland (Pierce *et al.* 2019) and NHS health boards in Scotland (Chambers and McKean 2017; Coutts 2014). OTHBMR is generally delivered over six to eight sessions in the person's own home, with or without a caregiver present, focusing on personalized and tailored memory strategies. There is a theme and purpose to each session, with information being repeated in subsequent sessions to encourage adoption of strategies.

Practical materials are introduced such as orientation clocks and white boards, to assist the person with their memory, and sessions are reinforced with printed information sheets, developed in partnership with people living with dementia, to support clarity of information and enhance understanding, and are presented in a positive way (DEEP 2013). The information sheets are referred to by the occupational therapist as the foundations of OTHBMR, where people are encouraged to learn the newly introduced tailored strategies and routines at the start of each weekly session, including a recap summary of the previous week that is rehearsed and emphasized with the occupational therapist. This summary is important as it further seeks to support and enable the person living with dementia to apply their new learning in their day-to-day life. This guides inclusion of the typical topic areas discussed in OTHBMR, as outlined below.

- *The memory book* is a customized resource where people are encouraged to record daily the day, date, month, year and information important to them, to help with orientation. It is also used to help the person plan via a 'To Do' list section. Key elements of the memory book are illustrated in Figure 14.1.

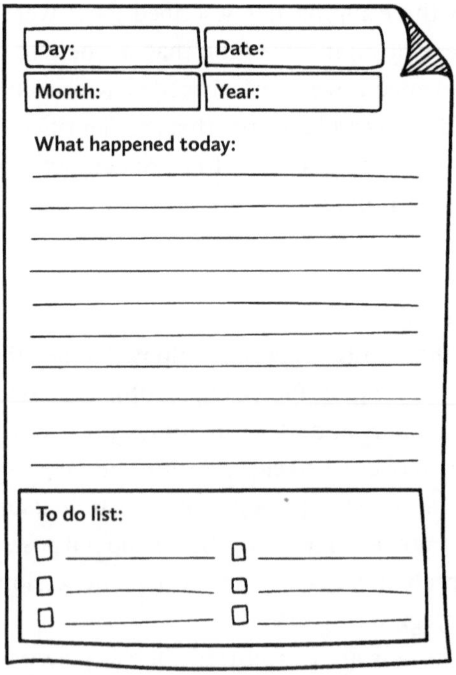

Figure 14.1. Example page from a memory book

The use of a memory book is often introduced in the first meeting between the person living with dementia and the occupational therapist, and is reinforced and supported throughout OTHBMR. Its use can help the person with their daily routines, supporting their memory for everyday events (episodic memory) as well as forward planning due to the structured layout of each page. The physical act of writing something down can reinforce routine, helping to pay attention to the information, and aids organization.

- *Remembering where you have put something* considers with the person strategies to organize their environment to enable and support their individual occupational participation in everyday activities, such as locating their house key or where to locate their passport. It requires emphasizing strategies that will support the person to undertake everyday tasks and in addition, enable good habits and routines needed to maintain these.

- *Remembering something you have to do* is about routine and the systems the person can use to enhance their independence in carrying out occupations identified as being important to them, as well as encouraging their safety when undertaking these (see Figure 14.2).

- *Remembering what people have told you* acknowledges that we can all have difficulty recalling what we have been told verbally, and encourages people to consider strategies that can support memory recall. It is tailored to what the person has highlighted as their main concern(s), for example answering the phone and having to act on the information.

- *Communicating* acknowledges the communication difficulties some people with dementia experience and the potential consequences this can have on their confidence, which may, in turn, result in the avoidance of previously valued occupations, such as ordering food in a restaurant or playing bowls. This session explores triggers or environments that can cause concern, and aims to encourage and co-create strategies that can help to reduce these, for example the use of assistance cards.

- *Keeping active* emphasizes the importance of looking after physical, emotional and cognitive health, and the interrelationship between these is considered as part of this session.

Discussion concentrates on sharing what 'being active' means to the person and how this can include diverse leisure pursuits, for example, photography, jigsaws or word searches, to more physical activities such as walking, golf or swimming. Key to this conversation is the value and importance placed by the person on activities they identify as being of importance to them.

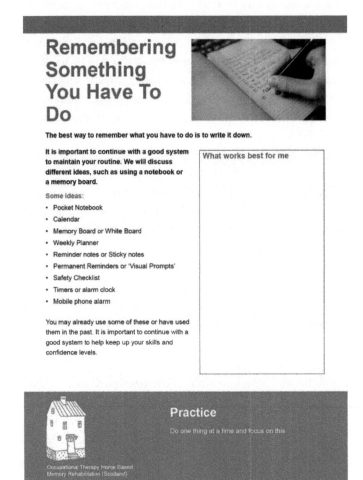

Figure 14.2. Information sheet: Remembering something you have to do

- *Relaxation* focuses on the need to prioritize relaxation time to maintain occupational balance. The need for this is likely to have been touched on in many sessions; however, there is an emphasis here on specific relaxation techniques, appropriate to the person and their needs. Relaxation is personal, with each of us having our preferred ways of practising this, for example, a soak in a bath, a breathing exercise, listening to music or going for a walk.

- *Out and about* is about accessing the person's local community and remaining socially connected to ensure their occupational engagement is maintained. There is an emphasis on habits and routines as well as using systems that encourage independence, for example arranging to swim on the same day each week. These sessions will include how to use transport and driving, if appropriate to the person.

Following the six to eight sessions of OTHBMR, a recommended review is carried out three months following completion, that is, three months after the final time the occupational therapist visits the person at home. This three-month review offers the person an opportunity to re-evaluate their co-created strategies, habits and routines, and to consider if further support and/or modification of approach is needed.

Evaluating OTHBMR in practice

One of the main drivers to deliver OTHBMR was for early post-diagnostic access to occupational therapy, when interventions can be particularly beneficial. However, of equal importance was to capture the impact of OTHBMR for the person living with dementia and their caregiver, and to begin to illustrate and build evidence of the effectiveness of occupational therapy. Initial and tentative evidence that supports the impact of OTHBMR includes the continued adoption of strategies to compensate for memory difficulties, used for up to two years following completion of this rehabilitation approach (McGrath and Passmore 2009). In addition, Coutts (2014) reported a decrease in the number of everyday memory difficulties people living with dementia experienced following OTHBMR, and people in the early stages of dementia were able to learn and retain new information (RCOT 2017).

To evaluate the ongoing impact of OTHBMR and to integrate and embed data collection as part of the everyday practice of occupational therapists in Scotland, a model for improvement (Langley *et al.* 2009) was used. This is supported by improvement tools such as project initiation documents, driver diagrams, measurement plans etc., with an equally strong focus on relational approaches such as local leadership, with an aim to create a shared vision for change. Initially OTHBMR was tested in one health board in Scotland (Coutts 2014) and then developed to a Scotland-wide national improvement project. As such, a national occupational therapy working group was established with the aim of enabling occupational therapists situated across each health board in Scotland to initially deliver OTHBMR to six people in each site. During the implementation phase, there were regular meetings to share progress, to explore what needed to be done differently and importantly, to gain agreement across Scotland on the adoption of the same outcome measures, including how these were to be used. This included discussion of outcome measures that had meaning to the person living with dementia, their caregiver, the occupational therapists and the wider multidisciplinary teams where they worked. The priority was always to keep the person at the centre of this improvement approach, whilst at the same time building the evidence base. As the work has evolved, and using feedback from people living with dementia, the occupational therapists are routinely collecting data.

At baseline, demographic information is recorded allowing the occupational therapist to understand their local population needs and to inform future developments. It was also important to have an up-to-date cognitive assessment to help inform the intervention. The number of everyday memory difficulties and memory strategies already in use are collected via checklists before OTHBMR begins, and are reviewed to measure impact at three months. Quality of life for both the person living with dementia and their caregiver is captured at baseline and review. Focusing on occupational performance, the Allen Cognitive Level Screen (ACLS) (Allen *et al.* 2007) is utilized at baseline and on review, and a goal-oriented occupational question is in development. Additional qualitative data is captured by way of case studies, use of emotional touchpoints, people's feedback and stories. Refer back to Chapter 13 to find out more about the ACLS, and Chapter 17, to find out more on evaluation in occupational therapy.

This work is ongoing and is complex in its design. It has been vital to ensure that the occupational therapists who participated in the improvement project, alongside people living with dementia, felt ownership of purpose, development and implementation. Local context in terms of geography (rural and urban areas) and experiences of practitioners, including the extent to which there is organizational support, can all vary. Agreement associated with outcome measures, both quantitative and qualitative, has needed to be reached, set within the overall aim of continued improvement. This work, therefore, is still to be fully evaluated and published; however, a qualitative research enquiry is currently being undertaken in one site in Scotland, focusing on the occupational therapists' experience of implementing OTHBMR prior to and during a pandemic. More generally, however, this national work has also led to wider conversations that help to support early access to occupational therapy services.

The integration of OTHBMR continues to evolve, and the occupational therapy work in Scotland has provided ongoing learning and collaboration, both nationally in the UK and internationally in the USA. We are also co-designing new methods to integrate technology to deliver OTHBMR, including the use of animation and short films to support the information sheets and memory strategies. As such, this improvement project has been a partnership between people living with dementia, their caregivers and occupational therapists in practice. To illustrate, an example of the delivery of OTHBMR, valuing the voice and experiences of people living with dementia, is outlined here.

THE LIVED EXPERIENCE: JULIA

Julia lived alone and had recently been diagnosed with Alzheimer's disease and vascular dementia. She had always been an independent person, but was concerned about her future because of her diagnoses. She was referred to occupational therapy by the local post-diagnostic service, who thought Julia would benefit from occupational therapy to learn practical coping strategies to help her stay connected with her local community. The occupational therapist met with Julia at home with her daughter, and it was agreed that OTHBMR should be adopted. The purpose of OTHBMR was explained to Julia, and her daughter and Julia were keen to participate in all areas of OTHBMR. The memory book was implemented at the beginning, with the additional sessions carried out in the order of Julia's priorities. Julia said she found all the sessions made her think about what she did day to day, and in particular, the benefits she identified from undertaking each of the weekly sessions:

- Memory book: 'I was initially very resistant to doing the memory book but agreed to give it a try. I soon realized I began to feel less stressed when asked a direct question, especially when my daughter phones and asks me what I have been doing, as I just need to look at my memory book.'
- Remembering something you have to do: 'I find my nightly checklist very reassuring. Before going to bed it reminds me to check my doors are locked and windows are closed, I've taken my medication and the next day's dinner is out of the freezer. I know if I see my checklist on my bedside table, I have done all the tasks, so can go to sleep and not have to check as I would have done before the checklist was introduced.'
- Remembering where you have put something: 'I often misplaced my house keys so found the suggestion of having these on a brightly coloured key chain with clip really helpful. I can now clip my keys onto a zip in my handbag or onto my belt loop and I keep them in my pocket when out. At home I keep them in a drawer and could easily locate them due to the brightly coloured key chain.'
- Out and about: 'When going out I could feel anxious due to my occasional word-finding difficulties. Being given a bespoke assistance card that I could show people to explain my difficulty has helped to give me reassurance. In addition, if I am going somewhere formal, for example, the bank or my dentist, I have started noting down what I want to say in a notebook, in advance, so I can refer to this.'
- Three-month review: 'The occupational therapist visited me at home three months after completion of the OTHBMR. I showed my occupational therapist photographs from a recent holiday, where I used ideas I gained from OTHBMR, which gave me confidence to go. I keep my photos in my memory book, and I continue to complete this each day, as it benefits me; my family and I would not be without it.'

Conclusion

In this chapter we have outlined the underpinning evidence, design and delivery, including ongoing evaluation, of OTHBMR. It is a growing area of interest as wider project evaluations begin to take place internationally and as circumstances alter, an example of which has been the COVID-19 pandemic, which has resulted in the online delivery of OTH-BMR, adding an additional strand to the existing evaluation pathways.

Irrespective of how it is delivered, OTHBMR remains an individualized and tailored occupational therapy rehabilitation programme for people living with dementia. The aspiration is that our work will continue to develop and spread so that as many people as possible can benefit from OTHBMR as a post-diagnostic intervention, upholding the right of people living with dementia to rehabilitation. In undertaking this work and in seeking to enhance our dementia practice, our advice is to ensure work such as this is undertaken collaboratively with others to take forward an idea, and to share the findings that emerge. Most important is to include and involve people living with dementia, which has been key to this work, as well as sharing and collaborating between passionate occupational therapists.

Reflective questions

1. On reading this chapter, what do you see as the potential benefits of OTHBMR, as an occupational therapy *post-diagnostic intervention*?
2. Use the memory book template in Figure 14.1 for a week, and then reflect on your occupations and routines during that time.
3. Consider an example of your practice-based experience or learning. What measures did you see adopted, and how were these used to evaluate the impact of occupational therapy practice?

References

Allen, C.K., Austin, S., David, S., Earhart, C., McCraith, D. and Riska-Williams, L. (2007) *Manual for the Allen Cognitive Level Screen (ACLS-5) and Large Allen Cognitive Level Screen (LACLS-5)*. Camarillo, CA: ACLS and LACLS Committee.

Cations, M., May, N., Crotty, M., Low, L.F., *et al.* (2020) 'Health professionals' perspectives on rehabilitation for people with dementia.' *The Gerontologist 60*, 3, 503–512.

Chambers, W. and McKean, A. (2017) 'When Opportunity Knocks: Developing and Delivering Evidence-based Post-diagnostic Interventions in Dementia: The National Occupational Therapy Experience in Scotland.' Presentation at Alzheimer Europe Conference: 'Care Today, Cure Tomorrow', 2–4 October, Berlin, Germany.

Clare, L. (2017) 'Rehabilitation for people living with dementia: A practical framework of positive support.' *PLoS MED 14*, 3, e1002245.

Clare, L., Kudlika, A., Oyebode, J.R., Jones, R.W., *et al.* (2019) 'Individual goal-oriented cognitive rehabilitation to improve everyday functioning for people with everyday dementia: A multicentre randomised controlled trial (the GREAT trial).' *International Journal of Geriatric Psychiatry 34*, 5, 709–721.

Coutts, E. (2014) *Allied Health Professionals Delivering Post-Diagnostic Support: Living Well with Dementia.* Edinburgh: Alzheimer Scotland. Accessed on 17/12/2021 at www.alzscot.org/sites/default/files/2019-07/AHP_Collaboration%20Document%20-%20Living%20with%20Dementia.pdf

DEEP (Dementia Engagement and Empowerment Project) (2013) 'Writing dementia-friendly information.' DEEP Guide. Accessed on 10/11/2021 at http://dementiavoices.org.uk/wp-content/uploads/2013/11/DEEP-Guide-Writing-dementia-friendly-information.pdf

Jogie, P., Rahja, M., van den Berg, M., Cations, M., Brown, S. and Laver, K. (2021) 'Goal setting for people with mild cognitive impairment or dementia in rehabilitation: A scoping review.' *Australian Occupational Therapy Journal 68*, 6, 563–592.

Langley, G.L., Moen, R.D., Nolan, K.M., Nolan, T.W., Norman, C.L. and Provost, L.P. (2009) *The Improvement Guide: A Practical Approach to Enhancing Organizational Performance* (2nd edn). San Francisco, CA: Jossey-Bass.

Low, L.F. and Laver, K. (eds) (2021) *Dementia Rehabilitation: Evidence-based Interventions and Clinical Recommendations.* London: Academic Press Elsevier.

Marshall, M. (2005) *Perspectives on Rehabilitation and Dementia.* London: Jessica Kingsley Publishers.

Maskill, L. and Tempest, S. (2017) *Neuropsychology for Occupational Therapists*: *Cognition in Occupational Performance* (4th edn). Oxford: John Wiley & Sons Ltd.

McGrath, M.P. (2013) *Promoting Safety in the Home: The Home Based Memory Rehabilitation Programme for Persons with Mild Alzheimer's Disease and Other Dementias.* London: The Health Foundation.

McGrath, M.P. and Passmore, P. (2009) 'Home Based Memory Rehabilitation Programme for persons with mild dementia.' *Irish Journal of Medical Science 178*, 8, S330.

NICE (National Institute for Health and Care Excellence) (2018) *Dementia: Assessment, Management and Support for People Living with Dementia and Their Carers.* NICE Guideline 97. London: NICE.

Pierce, M., Keogh, F., Teahan, A. and O'Shea, E. (2019) *Report of an Evaluation of the HSE's National Dementia Post-Diagnostic Support Grant Scheme.* Tullamore: National Dementia Office.

Ravn, M.B., Petersen, K.S. and Thuesen, J. (2019) 'Rehabilitation for people living with dementia: A scoping review of processes and outcomes.' *Journal of Aging Research 12*, 1–8.

RCOT (Royal College of Occupational Therapists) (2017) *Living not Existing: Putting Prevention at the Heart of Care for Older People in Scotland.* London: RCOT.

Sohlberg, M. and Mateer, C. (2001) *Cognitive Rehabilitation: An Integrative Neuropsy-chological Approach*. New York: Guilford Press.

WHO (World Health Organization) (2017) *Global Action Plan on the Public Health Response to Dementia 2017–2025*. Geneva: WHO. Accessed on 16/12/2021 at www. who.int/publications/i/item/global-action-plan-on-the-public-health-response -to-dementia-2017---2025

WHO (2020) 'Rehabilitation.' Geneva: WHO. Accessed on 20/12/2021 at www.who.int/ news-room/fact-sheets/detail/rehabilitation

Wilson, B. and Hughes, E. (1997) 'Coping with amnesia: The natural history of a com-pensatory memory system.' *Neuropsychological Rehabilitation 7*, 1, 43–56.

CHAPTER 15

Journeying through Dementia
An Occupation-Based Group Approach for Individuals Following Diagnosis

Claire Craig, Helen Fisher, Ashleigh Gray and Elaine Hunter

Learning outcomes
By the end of this chapter, you will have the opportunity to:

▸ Understand the value of a community-based group intervention for people living with dementia
▸ Gain insight into the key role of occupational therapists in working with people living with dementia following diagnosis
▸ Recognize and reflect on the importance of intersectorial and interdisciplinary working.

Introduction

This chapter describes a post-diagnostic occupational therapy group programme called 'Journeying through Dementia' (Mountain and Craig 2012). The programme, co-designed with people living with dementia, provides an opportunity for individuals to develop the skills and techniques necessary to maintain occupational engagement as the condition progresses. We highlight the central role occupational therapists play in working with individuals, post-diagnosis, and the value of group work and community-based approaches.

This chapter begins by sharing the voices of people living with dementia who describe the value of occupation. These accounts are followed by a brief overview of UK policy as we consider what the broader evidence tells us about existing approaches to support individuals and their families. The Journeying through Dementia intervention is then described, and we detail how the principles underpinning the programme relate both to the broader evidence and to the core philosophy of occupational therapy. We conclude by reflecting on some of the key learning from implementing the group.

The key message we hope that you will take away is the value of occupation-based group work that recognizes the strengths of individuals and the community resources that people living with dementia can draw on and contribute to.

Context

As other parts of this book have highlighted, dementia is a long-term, degenerative, neurological condition that currently impacts on the lives of 10 million individuals and their families in Europe (Vernooij-Dassen *et al.* 2021). The cognitive changes occurring as a consequence of dementia can affect almost every area of occupational functioning. Activities of daily living that allow individuals to live independently can be severely compromised as a result of difficulties in short-term memory, sequencing and planned purposeful movement (praxis). Communication problems (dysphasia and anomia) can make social participation challenging (Maki and Endo 2018).

What people with dementia tell us

Whilst there is burgeoning literature about dementia, much of this has been presented through a biomedical lens with an emphasis on dementia as a disease and a focus on cognition (Vernooij-Dassen *et al.* 2021). This picture is gradually shifting as people living with dementia share their experiences. Advocacy groups comprising people with dementia include the Scottish Dementia Working Group (SDWG), the Dementia Engagement and Empowerment Project (DEEP Network) and the Dementia Advocacy and Support Network International (DASNI), leading the way in challenging negative stereotypes associated with the condition and sharing ways that people can live well.

As occupational therapists we have much to learn from people living with dementia and their families, and their descriptions of the central role that occupation plays in promoting wellbeing. Accounts from people with dementia highlight how meaningful occupation supports engagement, promoting mental wellbeing and providing individuals with an aim and an outlet for self-expression. People living with dementia have described the value of occupation in finding a purpose in life (Perkins *et al.* 2016).

We hear accounts of people speaking about the importance of leisure and recreational activities as vehicles for self-expression, as embodied in the following quote: 'Our experiences during leisure mean something important to each of us. Leisure allows us to continue to express who we are and what we value about ourselves by using our unique skills and abilities gained over our lifetimes' (quoted in Hounam 2011, p.3). People with dementia speak of how engaging in occupation provides a structure to the day and a focus, and the importance of 'Keeping busy, it doesn't matter what it is. At the start of the day, I look forward to what I am doing next and I am working doing everything I can possibly do' (Matt, SDWG member, quoted in Weaks *et al.* 2012, p.16).

Whilst there is no denying that dementia can have a significant impact on every aspect of occupational functioning, a number of people living with dementia, including Agnes Houston, Wendy Mitchell, James McKillop and Christine Bryden, through a range of publications, have highlighted that dementia has on occasion led to the development of new interests and occupations. In the words of Agnes Houston, 'I believe I have a duty to let the public know that a diagnosis of dementia is not the end, but the beginning of a new life' (quoted in Weaks *et al.* 2012, p.8).

Significantly, people with dementia highlight the value of peer support, of people coming together to share their experiences and make sense of living with the condition: 'Coming here was one of the best things I ever did, because all these people were in the same boat as me doing something useful and this is probably why I still come, because I am doing something useful' (David, SDWG member, quoted in Weaks *et al.* 2012, p.11).

These social networks are vital as above all they enable individuals to maintain community connectedness, and also to practice and continue to engage in meaningful occupation.

The value of occupation

Kitwood (1997) viewed engagement in occupation as central to being connected and engaged in life, a core facet of personhood. A body of evidence to support the relationship between wellbeing and occupation exists (Mok *et al.* 2007). An early systematic review of over 3000 papers by Egan, Hobson and Fearing (2006) concluded that there was clear evidence to support the relationship between enabling occupation and quality of life for people with dementia. This was also a key theme identified by Wolverson, Clarke and Moniz-Cook (2016) in their systematic review of the literature about the factors that enable people with dementia to live positively with the condition.

Indeed, occupational therapists have an important role to play in supporting individuals living with dementia to continue to engage in meaningful occupation. Preventative actions, adopting a proactive approach to health and wellbeing, is much more likely to enable enhanced outcomes for people with dementia and their families as opposed to suggestions made in times of crisis when making adjustments to the environment.

One of the challenges is that the biomedical model dominates many services, and consequently these can sometimes be at odds with occupational therapists' person-centred holistic approach. In one Australian study, Bennett, Shand and Liddle (2011) found that occupational therapists working with people living with dementia spent most of their time undertaking assessments, providing equipment and offering advice regarding environmental modifications. In a study undertaken in Ireland, McGrath and O'Callaghan (2014) similarly found that there was limited attention given to occupational participation, with emphasis again placed on the provision of assistive devices and environmental modifications to the home. This is in spite of a growing evidence base that tells us of the importance of early, home and community-focused interventions (Quinn *et al.* 2016).

Dementia policy globally has focused on delivering a timely diagnosis. In the UK, as early as 2013, the G8 Summit on Dementia prioritized early intervention and care in the community and in people's own homes. A number of key policies support this approach. For instance, *Connecting People, Connecting Support* (Alzheimer Scotland 2017, 2020) was the national framework for transforming the contribution of allied health professionals to supporting people living with dementia and those who support them. Its aspiration is that people have better access to allied health professionals, regardless of age or place of residence, from pre-diagnosis to diagnosis and throughout their illness.

Approaches that focus on the strengths and resources individuals and communities possess sit well with occupational therapy's enabling and empowering philosophy. The community is where many occupations are enacted, and over the last decade a significant international movement has focused on the creation of age-friendly and dementia-friendly cities. These are seen as places 'that maximise independence through collaboration with diverse community stakeholders (Turner and Morken 2016)' and which 'shift the narrative from deficit and burden to contribution and inclusion to mitigate against stigma, prejudice and discrimination' (Raham and Swaffer 2018, p.132). These initiatives reflect a concurrent movement that has sought to equip people living with dementia with strategies to manage their condition. This self-management approach has been in existence for some time for individuals living with other long-term conditions such as diabetes and heart disease (Lorig and Holman 2003).

However, the challenge is that the model of self-management proposed by Lorig and Holman (2003) was aimed at long-term physical health conditions as opposed to individuals managing cognitive change, and for some time there was a lack of clarity as to what self-management meant for people living with dementia (Mountain 2006).

We were inspired to collaborate together and change this. We wanted to integrate the key principles of the original research by Mountain and Craig (2012) and recent work by Wright *et al.* (2019) on self-management in dementia and implement them. We took a practical and pragmatic approach guided by improvement science (Langley *et al.* 2009), and worked in partnership with the original researcher, a designer and local occupational therapy services to implement Journey through Dementia in a local context. We were able to draw on the experiences of the SDWG, one of the first peer-to-peer campaign groups to be established, and the inspiration behind Journeying through Dementia throughout the project timeline from 2006 to 2020 (see Figure 15.1).

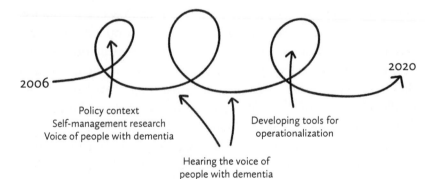

Figure 15.1. Project timeline

Journeying through Dementia: an occupational therapy group intervention

Journeying through Dementia is an occupation-based intervention that aims to support people with dementia at an early stage of their dementia journey to engage in meaningful activities and maintain community connectedness. Claire, one of the authors of this chapter, undertook a research enquiry to build understanding of what people living with the condition felt they would find useful post-diagnosis. Individuals who took part in the research described the value they attached to continued participation in everyday occupations and in new learning. Throughout all the co-creation activities people with dementia took part in, the message was clear – individuals wanted to meet other people living with dementia to share their experiences, learn from the experiences of others and to develop strategies to enable them to live well with the condition.

The output of the research was an evidence-based group intervention named Journeying through Dementia. At the heart of the intervention is a two-hour weekly group meeting that is held in the community and facilitated by occupational therapists. During this 8- to 12-week programme the occupational therapist also visits the person at home up to three times to ensure that the group is customized to meet the needs of its members and is enabling them to meet their own goals.

Group work enables participants to explore topics and concepts. Through a process of exchange and guidance participants have the opportunity to reflect on the range of activities they take part in, to talk about their experiences and share strategies they have found useful in overcoming the challenges that living with a diagnosis of dementia can bring. They have the opportunity to enact their skills in the community through engagement in a series of out-of-venue activities (for example, cafes, public libraries, markets). Here, ideas or techniques and skills discussed in sessions can be put into practice, and participants have the opportunity to test out ideas and rehearse skills, to step outside their comfort zones to transform the discussion that has occurred within group sessions into a lived experience.

The programme is underpinned by a number of key principles, cognisant with the philosophy of occupational therapy, which distinguish it from other post-diagnostic support programmes. The focus throughout is on adaptation and grading to maximize participation in occupation. Rather than focusing on dementia as a disease within the programme, dementia is viewed as a constant process of change and adaptation. As a person's journey through dementia progresses, different strategies will be required. Finding ways to modify or adapt the way that activities and routines are performed, the person and their family are supported to maximize participation and promote continued wellbeing throughout their journey with the condition. Sessions are structured around information sharing by the facilitator, but great emphasis is placed on discussion topics that encourage participants to share strategies to help mitigate some of the symptoms of dementia. This helps position individuals as experts at managing their condition, and reflects a strengths-based approach where participants' abilities are key resources (see Figure 15.2).

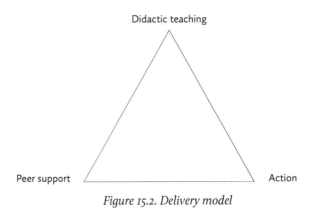

Figure 15.2. Delivery model

Emphasis throughout is placed on doing rather than simply talking about strategies and challenges. Individuals are given the opportunity to put ideas into practice, either within the group or through organized out-of-venue activities, away from the home and in the local community. This helps to build confidence and also encourages active problem-solving. The community is seen as a place where skills are enacted, and where individuals can access a wide range of resources to support roles, maintain and develop relationships and to experience enjoyable leisure activities that support wellbeing.

Journeying through Dementia recognizes that each group will be different, and is therefore comprised of a menu of topics that participants can choose from. In this way the intervention is customized to meet the needs of individuals. This also helps to build self-efficacy through promoting active choice and decision-making. Individual sessions also offer the opportunity to address particular goals group members may have, and permit further levels of customization.

Finally, the programme offers hope by challenging some of the preconceptions that exist in relation to what people with dementia can achieve.

Journeying through Dementia: co-designing the materials

We all recognized the importance of creating high-quality materials that communicated to those attending and were also valued by those facilitating the programme. The Journeying through Dementia facilitation materials went through five iterations following co-design workshops between 2017 and 2019, and were described by the occupational therapists as 'ageless, the design is not stigmatizing' and 'something that inspires hope and creates excitement' (see Figure 15.3). Co-design and co-production is something that occupational therapists do naturally, working with diverse people and groups to develop solutions.

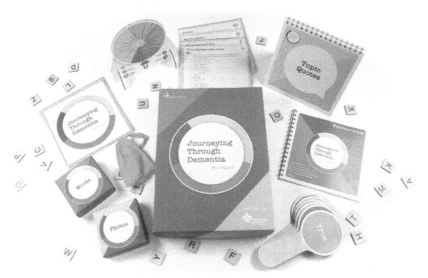

Figure 15.3. Journeying Through Dementia group facilitation kit (www.jtd.org.uk)

The components of the materials are summarized as:

- *Photographs* are used during the groups as prompts and ways to share what is meaningful to individuals. Participants particularly enjoyed the use of photographs within the group, noting that they were relatable.
- *True and false paddles* are used to make the quizzes more interactive, and allow people to express themselves without having to speak up if they do not wish to.
- The *word cards* work in a similar way – participants can choose from a range of emotions, questions and prompts to express how they feel about something.
- The *spinner* adds another level of interactivity, and helps with decision-making within the group.
- The *topic quotes* allow for other perspectives from other people with dementia on a particular topic, to spark discussions.
- *Scrabble letters* are used in different ways as prompts; having objects that are familiar, such as Scrabble letters, helped people to relate and engage.
- The Journeying through Dementia *sign* helps participants navigate a space and feel confident that they are in the right place; it also sets the scene and offers a level of familiarity every week.

These were designed to encourage group participation and allow individuals to develop relationships with those in the group through understanding what was meaningful to them, and helping each other to develop strategies to continue to do what they love and maintain community connectedness.

Journeying through Dementia: the occupational therapists' insights

Journeying through Dementia was initially implemented across two sites in Scotland, and an evaluation of the impact of the intervention was undertaken by occupational therapists using a number of tools and measures, including the Quality of Life in Alzheimer's Disease (QOL-AD) scale. Each site also undertook additional assessments, as per local guidance and practices. Demographic data was recorded, and an occupation-based, goal-oriented question was included to measure personal experience and provide an occupation-focused outcome measure. A Likert scale was used in line with Scotland's national review of post-diagnostic support, to consider how helpful participants had found the intervention, with an opportunity to add any supporting comments. Participants were also asked for weekly feedback on their experience of the group, and therapists were interviewed by Ashleigh, one of the authors of this chapter. This involved gaining therapist understanding of facilitating the intervention, and insights were used to inform and guide the development of the next phase of work.

Here are some of the insights the participants shared:

- The group work element of the programme was frequently commented on by participants, who valued the opportunity for open communication. They fed back that they felt they 'were helping one another being on the same wave length' and feeling 'very comfortable' as they could speak openly in a non-judgemental atmosphere. Within the group setting they were able to draw on the experiences of others, sharing their resourcefulness as well as being a group resource.

- The value of the group as a place for learning and rehearsal of skills for participants and experimentation was clear. The opportunity to take what was learned in the group into the community enabled individuals to build confidence and create community connectedness for ongoing occupational engagement. Group members could and did engage in group problem-solving, identifying potential resources they could draw on moving forwards.

- The skills required by the occupational therapists to create the conditions to enable this to happen in the group should not be underestimated. The therapists succeeded in creating a safe space where participants could openly share their thoughts, feelings and experiences of living with dementia and the challenges they faced when engaging in valued occupations. They achieved the balance between creating an environment that was both relaxed and fun but that also used gentle reinforcement and collaboration to maximize inclusion for all group members.

- Recruitment of appropriate individuals to the group was particularly important, and it was challenging to identify people in the early stages of their dementia journey as many services are focused on addressing the needs of people whose dementia is more advanced. In order to overcome this challenge, facilitators shared information leaflets and offered to speak further with healthcare teams and referrers about the intervention. The facilitators agreed that in order to facilitate the intervention and target this support in the most effective way possible, pre-screening was a vital aspect of identifying those for whom the intervention might be most suitable. Ensuring that potential referrers understood the purpose and aims of the group was important, and the facilitators sought to gain information from several sources in order to identify people who may benefit from the programme.
- The facilitators agreed that Journeying through Dementia is a high-quality resource that provides a structure to each session, but that also offers flexibility in being able to adapt to the needs of the participants and incorporate one-to-one and out-of-venue sessions to support programme delivery. The wealth of themes and resources available, that are also adaptable to the needs of the group, is vitally important in providing the customization to the participants' needs. The group materials were carefully considered and professionally presented; the value placed in the resource articulates the value offered to the participants.
- The facilitators were initially apprehensive regarding delivering a programme that was so flexible and not planned from the outset; however, provisions such as the topic wheel and booklets proved beneficial to support initial discussions around selecting appropriate sessions, and this process became easier as relationships were established and the participants identified topics they wanted to look at in more detail.

Conclusion

This chapter has offered an overview of a community-based group programme for individuals recently diagnosed with dementia. The programme, named Journeying through Dementia, focuses on enabling individuals to develop skills and techniques to adapt activities in order to continue to engage in those occupations that are so central to their quality of life.

We began the chapter with reflections from people living with the condition on the importance of occupation before describing the creation of the Journeying through Dementia rehabilitation intervention, and how this focus on early intervention relates to the broader evidence and policy framework. The chapter briefly touched on the design of the materials before sharing some of the experiences of people with dementia and occupational therapists involved in the delivery of the programme.

We hope, above all, that this chapter has offered you a glimpse of the value of an occupation-based group programme that can be customized to the needs of individuals attending this, and that we have given you the confidence to revisit your group work skills in the context of working with individuals living with dementia.

Reflective questions

After reading this chapter we would like you to:

1. Take note of how many occupations you perform in group contexts. Write down, draw and reflect on all the things you value about being in a group.
2. Take time to explore your community, and identify all the opportunities and resources that the community holds for people living with dementia.
3. Think of all the ways that the community where you live could benefit from input from individuals living with dementia.

References

Alzheimer Scotland (2017) *Connecting People, Connecting Support: Transforming the Allied Health Professions' Contribution to Supporting People Living with Dementia in Scotland, 2017–2020.* Edinburgh: Alzheimer Scotland. Accessed on 25/04/2022 at www.alzscot.org/sites/default/files/images/0002/7355/AHP_Report_2017_WEB.pdf

Alzheimer Scotland (2020) *Connecting People, Connecting Support in Action: An Impact Report on Transforming the Allied Health Professions' Contribution to Supporting People Living with Dementia in Scotland.* Edinburgh: Alzheimer Scotland. Accessed on 25/04/2022 at www.alzscot.org/sites/default/files/2020-03/Connecting%20 People%20Connecting%20Support%20in%20action%20report.pdf

Bennett, S., Shand, S. and Liddle, J. (2011) 'Occupational therapy practice in Australia with people with dementia: A profile in need of change.' *Australian Occupational Therapy Journal 58,* 155–163.

Egan, M., Hobson, S. and Fearing, V. (2006) 'Dementia and occupation: A review of the literature.' *Canadian Journal of Occupational Therapy 73,* 3, 132–140.

Hounam, B. (2011) *By Us for Us: Guide Celebrating Life through Leisure.* Waterloo, ON: Research Institute for Aging.

Kitwood, T. (1997) *Dementia Reconsidered: The Person Comes First.* Buckingham: Open University Press.

Langley, G.L., Moen, R.D., Nolan, K.M., Nolan, T.W., Norman, C.L. and Provost, L.P. (2009) *The Improvement Guide: A Practical Approach to Enhancing Organizational Performance* (2nd edn). San Francisco, CA: Jossey-Bass.

Lorig, K.R. and Holman, H. (2003) 'Self-management education: History, definition, outcomes, and mechanisms.' *Annals of Behavioral Medicine 26,* 1, 1–7.

Maki, Y. and Endo, H. (2018) 'The contribution of occupational therapy to building a dementia-positive community.' *British Journal of Occupational Therapy 81,* 10, 566–570.

McGrath, M. and O'Callaghan, C. (2014) 'Occupational therapy and dementia care: A survey of practice in the Republic of Ireland.' *Australian Occupational Therapy Journal 61,* 2, 92–101.

Mok, E., Lai, C.K.Y., Wong, F.L.F. and Wan, P. (2007) 'Living with early-stage dementia: The perspective of older Chinese people.' *Journal of Advanced Nursing 59,* 591–600.

Mountain, G. (2006) 'Self-management for people with early dementia: An exploration of concepts and supporting evidence.' *Dementia 5,* 3, 429–446.

Mountain, G. and Craig, C. (2012) 'What should be in a self-management programme for people with early dementia?' *Aging and Mental Health 16,* 5, 576–583.

Perkins, R., Hill, L., Daley, S., Chappell, M. and Rennison, J. (2016) *Continuing to Be Me – Recovering a Life with a Diagnosis of Dementia.* Nottingham: ImROC.

Quinn, C., Toms, G., Jones, C., Brand, A., *et al.* (2016) 'A pilot randomized controlled trial of a self-management group intervention for people with early-stage dementia (The SMART study).' *International Psychogeriatrics 28,* 5, 787–800. doi:10.1017/S1041610215002094

Raham, S. and Swaffer, K. (2018) 'Assets-based approaches and dementia-friendly communities.' *Dementia 17,* 2, 131–137.

Turner, N. and Morken, L. (2016) *Better Together: A Comparative Analysis of Age-friendly and Dementia-friendly Communities.* Accessed on 14/07/2022 at www.aarp.org/livable-communities/network-age-friendly-communities/info-2016/dementia-friendly-communities.html

Vernooij-Dassen, M., Moniz-Cook, E., Verhey, F., Chattat, R., *et al.* (2021) 'Bridging the divide between biomedical and psychosocial approaches in dementia research: The 2019 INTERDEM manifesto.' *Aging & Mental Health 25,* 2, 206–212. doi:10.1080/13607863.2019.1693968

Weaks, D., Wilkinson, H., Houston, A. and McKillop, J. (2012) *Perspectives on Ageing with Dementia.* York: Joseph Rowntree Foundation.

Wolverson, E.L., Clarke, C. and Moniz-Cook, E.D. (2016) 'Living positively with dementia: A systematic review and synthesis of the qualitative literature.' *Aging & Mental
Health 20*, 7, 676–699.

Wright, J., Foster, A., Cooper, C., Sprange, K., *et al.* (2019) 'Study protocol for a randomised controlled trial assessing the clinical and cost-effectiveness of the Journeying through Dementia (JtD) intervention compared to usual care.' *BMJ Open
9*, e029207. doi:10.1136/bmjopen-2019-029207

CHAPTER 16

Working with People with Dementia and their Caregivers

Tailored Activity Program (TAP) and Care of People with Dementia in their Environments (COPE) in Action

Caroline Kate Keefe, Alison McKean, Jill Cigliana,
Kari Burch and Catherine Verrier Piersol

Learning outcomes

By the end of this chapter, you will have the opportunity to:

▸ Describe the models that inform two evidence-based interventions, the Tailored Activity Program (TAP) and Care of People with Dementia in their Environments (COPE)
▸ Identify common behavioural symptoms of dementia and the treatment outcomes of TAP and COPE
▸ Apply the treatment principles of TAP and COPE to case studies, and explore implementation in practice.

Introduction

As the population reaches the ages of 65 to 85, the morbidity of Alzheimer's disease and related dementias increases exponentially (Alzheimer's Association 2021). The World Health Organization (WHO) (2020) reports approximately 50 million people are living with dementia, and estimates that this number will increase to 82 million by 2030 and 152 million by 2050. As cognitive function declines, people living with dementia require support to perform everyday tasks and activities. In addition, behavioural symptoms impact the lives of family caregivers, increase care costs, the risk for placement in care homes, and hospitalizations, and correlate with mortality (Gitlin, Jacobs and Earland 2010; Sivananthan and McGrail 2016). Behavioural symptoms most troubling to families include apathy, agitation, irritability, sleep and appetite changes, mood disturbances, disinhibition, hallucinations, resistance to care and wandering (Mukherjee *et al.* 2017). A wide body of evidence shows that commonly prescribed antipsychotic medications are ineffective in managing behaviours and associated with poor health outcomes. Evidentiary support demonstrates that non-pharmacological interventions are effective in managing behavioural symptoms with people living with dementia (Fraker *et al.* 2014; Gitlin *et al.* 2010).

Occupational therapy can meet this need through evidence-based, non-pharmacological interventions that promote caregiver knowledge and skills in customized strategies, thereby optimizing function and quality of life for all involved (Fraker *et al.* 2014). In response to the monumental need for non-pharmacological intervention and the substantive body of evidence that supports occupational therapy's role in service delivery, this chapter describes two evidence-based interventions – the Tailored Activity Program (TAP) and the Care of Persons with Dementia in their Environments (COPE) – both designed to support community-dwelling people living with dementia and their family caregivers.

Description of need and dementia care best practices

The role of occupational therapy in dementia care includes assessment of preserved capacities and occupational performance in the person living with dementia, the physical and social environment, and the caregiver's needs and abilities. Caregivers play a critical role in dementia care, as they offer information regarding life history, habits, routines, roles, culture and preferences (Fraker *et al.* 2014). Limited knowledge about disease progression, lack of contextual support and unexpected shifting roles contribute to the rise in stress and burden associated with caregiving (Gitlin *et al.* 2008). Further, caregivers often overestimate the abilities of the person living with dementia (Burch and Burch 2021; Piersol *et al.* 2016). Evidence supports intervention for the dyad – the person living with dementia and their caregiver – as both are at risk of poor health and quality of life (Alzheimer's Association 2021). Best practices in dementia care include evidence and theoretical models to guide clinical practice.

Models that inform TAP and COPE

Several models guide clinical reasoning applied in the delivery of TAP and COPE:

- The *Cognitive Disabilities Model* (CDM) (McCraith and Earhart 2018) characterizes the typical patterns of cognitive function in six hierarchical levels (the Allen Cognitive Levels Screen (ACLS)) based on global cognition functions and environmental characteristics that support the performance of desired tasks as independently and safely as possible, by identifying prescribed capacities and optimizing functional performance by using the correct level of caregiver cues and support.
- The *Stress Process Model* (Pearlin *et al.* 1981) posits that personal resources (self-competence, mastery and self-efficacy) and social supports (emotional, instrumental, perceived and structural) are protective factors that buffer the negative impacts of stress. Interventions targeting skill-building in the caregiver and identifying support mechanisms reduce the stress and burden of caregiving.
- The *Competence-Environmental Press Framework* (Lawton and Nahemow 1974) explains the influence of the physical environment on an individual's behaviour. When the demand or press of the environment is too high (for example, too much noise or cluttered space), performance becomes subpar and behavioural symptoms may be triggered. Interventions that teach caregivers how to modify the environment and their own approach optimize performance and reduce the potential for behavioural symptoms in the person living with dementia.
- The *Transtheoretical Model* (Gitlin and Rose 2016) explains behaviour change in stages, based on the individual's readiness or intention to change what they do. The model posits that behaviour change does not occur until the individual is ready,

so treatment must meet the individual's level of readiness. Caregivers knowledgeable about dementia who exhibit a readiness to try new strategies will benefit more from different types of education and training than those with little knowledge of dementia or limited readiness to change. The intervention provided must meet the caregiver where there is readiness to implement strategies to help them move through the stages of change.

In the delivery of TAP and COPE, these models help explain the intersection between preserved capacities and the demands of the environment and task, which impacts dementia-related behaviours and performance in the person living with dementia, and therefore guides the occupational therapist's clinical reasoning. Furthermore, the occupational therapist provides caregiver education and training at their level of readiness to implement new knowledge and skills, including simplifying tasks and communication strategies and modifying the environment for success.

Evidence-based interventions for people with dementia and their caregivers

A review of the literature elucidates that occupational therapy interventions that support the person living with dementia and the caregiver have evolved from the Skills2Care® program (previously the Environmental Skill-building Program) (Gitlin *et al.* 2001; Gitlin, Jacobs and Earland 2010), TAP (Gitlin *et al.* 2008, 2018) and COPE (Fortinsky *et al.* 2020; Gitlin *et al.* 2010). Skills2Care® educates caregivers about dementia and behavioural symptoms, teaches techniques for taking care of self, and uses a problem-solving approach to address caregiver-identified problems. TAP is a program for caregivers that includes an assessment of the person living with dementia to identify preserved capabilities and interests, from which activity prescriptions provide caregivers with specific strategies to promote activity engagement. Finally, the COPE program draws from Skills2Care® and TAP to include the components of both programs. In this chapter we describe TAP and COPE, and provide case studies to demonstrate how each intervention is applied in practice.

Treatment principles of TAP and COPE

Both interventions have clearly defined treatment principles (see Table 16.1) that are immutable, and so must be followed to maintain fidelity (that is, the extent to which the delivery of the intervention sufficiently adheres to protocols originally developed to produce the same outcome and effectiveness for clients). Formal education and training are required regarding the theoretical foundations of TAP and COPE, intervention and delivery, and methods for adaptation to specific practice settings.

To maintain fidelity of the intervention, it is essential that services be delivered in a client-centred fashion, individualized to the pre-served capacities of the person living with dementia and focused on the caregiver's goals and expectations rather than on priorities or goals imposed by the practitioner. Through collaboration with the client and caregiver, the practitioner guides the caregiver to a deeper understanding of the disease process and how to alter their expectations (task, environment and communication style), and matches the abilities of the person living with dementia to the demands of the task, all of which mitigate everyday care challenges.

Table 16.1. TAP and COPE treatment principles

Treatment principle	Description
Client-centred and family-directed	Targets problems or activities that the caregiver identifies as important
Customized to interests and preferences	Education, strategies and activities reflect the interests and preferences of the dyad
Culturally relevant	Education, strategies and activities are consistent with roles, habits and family values
Problem-solving oriented	Uses problem-solving and mind mapping to identify strategies and activities
Active engagement	Employs experiential learning through doing approaches

In contrast, characteristics that are mutable include the dosage of the intervention sessions and when intervention components are provided. Adjustments to the protocol must be made to meet the caregiver's needs, adjusted to the abilities of the person living with dementia, and comply with the requirements of the service delivery setting.

Tailored Activity Program (TAP)

TAP is an evidence-based occupational therapy intervention that facilitates activity engagement, reduces behavioural symptoms in the person living with dementia and improves caregiver self-efficacy (Gitlin *et al.* 2008). The program teaches caregivers to set up and engage the person living with dementia in familiar and meaningful activities that are modified based on the capacities of the person (Gitlin *et al.* 2008, 2009). Caregivers learn to simplify the environment, task and strategies for communication.

TAP includes eight sessions over three phases – assessment, implementation and generalization. The assessment reveals preserved capacities, physical ability and limitations, and activity interests in the person living with dementia. Assessment of caregiver knowledge, readiness to implement activities and communication style, along with environmental characteristics, provide a comprehensive pallet from which to design activities. Drawing on assessment findings, the practitioner, the person living with dementia and their caregiver collaborate to identify appropriate activities, and the practitioner creates up to three activity prescriptions. With instruction, practice and feedback, the caregiver implements the activity prescriptions with the person living with dementia. The generalization of activity strategies (for example, task simplification, environmental modifications and cuing techniques) to other daily activities and the process for simplifying strategies as the disease progresses complete the program.

TAP demonstrates cross-cultural relevance, and is currently delivered in Australia, Brazil, Chile, Hong Kong, Italy, Russia, Scotland and the USA. In Brazil, a randomized trial of TAP implementation found significant reductions in the number, frequency and intensity of behavioural symptoms and caregiver distress, as well as improvements in the quality of life for people living with dementia and their caregivers (Novelli *et al.* 2018). In addition, a national improvement project led by Scotland's leading dementia charity, Alzheimer Scotland, began in 2012 that aims to translate the TAP into local practice (Reid 2014). TAP was selected as it aligned to the *Delivering Integrated Dementia Care: The 8 Pillars of*

Community Support approach developed by Alzheimer Scotland (2012), the aim of which is to build the community resilience of people living with dementia and their caregivers to enable them to remain part of their community for as long as possible.

Following consultation with the developers of this intervention, over 40 occupational therapists have now been trained in TAP since 2012. This has contributed to the development of an ongoing occupational therapy community of practice that shares experiences and learning connected to the delivery of this intervention, which includes the vital partnership working with caregivers. This improvement approach therefore commits to growing and evolving the evidence base for TAP in Scotland, in parallel translating evidence with practice. An example illustrating the implementation of TAP is highlighted below.

TAP CASE STUDY: ALAN AND MARY

Alan lives with his wife Mary. Alan was diagnosed with Alzheimer's disease at the age of 73. His medical history includes hypertension. Several years ago, Alan turned over the operations of the family business to his son-in-law. His family noticed that Alan was not adapting well to retirement and was becoming increasingly isolated and not going out of the house. He was referred to occupational therapy to address limited meaningful activities and a loss of self-esteem.

The occupational therapist completed a range of assessments including the Large Allan Cognitive Levels Screen (LACLS) and the Timed UP and Go (TUG) test. Both are key assessments integral to the TAP intervention. In the TUG it was noted that Alan was able to transfer safely and walk up to 15 minutes with a steady pace, utilizing his walking stick. Mary had concerns that he might fall due to his age, and discouraged him from walking outside alone. This led to conflict, as Alan did not want to be viewed 'as a child'. It was difficult to identify his hobbies or interests, as Alan's identity was intricately tied to his work. Mary felt Alan would be less irritable at home if he worked in the family business where he felt valued and productive. Mary also recognized that she needed time at home alone to do housework. Together with the occupational therapist, Alan and Mary identified the following goals:

1. Walk around his town where he is well known and will have opportunities to interact socially with others.
2. Work in the family business, sanding, varnishing and assembling garden furniture.

The couple participated in ten home visits and one workplace visit. An education approach addressed the importance of physical activity to maintain Alan's strength and promote his physical wellbeing (targeting his preserved capabilities rather than his limitations). Activity prescriptions were completed to achieve each goal. Alan's family agreed it would be beneficial for him to walk the familiar ten-minute journey to the family business, and his son-in-law was happy to have Alan attend the business a couple of times a week to assist with assembling garden furniture.

The workplace visit focused on task analysis of furniture assembly and matching task demand to Alan's capacities. Assembling chairs from pre-cut pieces was identified as a task that Alan could complete alongside another worker. Two workstations were set up next to each other, allowing Alan to mirror the other worker whilst enjoying workplace chats; thus, task and environmental modifications allowed Alan the satisfaction of contributing to the family business in a tangible way whilst maintaining social connection.

Through activity engagement, Alan was visibly more cheerful during the later occupational therapy visits, and talked about his work in the family business with pride. Mary was pleased to share that Alan was less irritable on the days that he was at home with her.

Care of Persons with Dementia in their Environment (COPE)

COPE includes six to ten sessions in the home across three phases – assessment, implementation and generalization. As with TAP, the assessment phase involves evaluating the person living with dementia, the caregiver and the environment. Practitioners perform a structured interview with the caregiver to determine and prioritize their self-identified problems. The practitioner uses active listening and poses probing questions to gain an insight into why the target problems are challenging for the caregiver.

The intervention phase addresses the caregiver-identified problems, including the implementation of an activity, drawing from TAP. The practitioner guides the caregiver through a structured problem-solving and mind-mapping process to elucidate root causes or triggers of the problem and potential solutions. COPE prescriptions are created, delivered and practised with the caregiver. Approaches to this process are adjusted to the readiness of the caregiver to implement strategies. As in TAP, the modification and generalization of strategies is the focus of the generalization phase to facilitate caregiver confidence. Here is an example illustrating the implementation of COPE:

COPE CASE STUDY: ROSE AND RANDALL

Rose lives with her husband Randall. Rose is 78 years old, and was diagnosed with Alzheimer's disease two years ago, with comorbidities of anxiety and depression. They were referred to a local COPE programme by emergency medical services due to Rose's repeated falls.

The assessment process revealed that Rose was unsafe to be alone at home, able to engage in repetitive activities, and able to notice objects directly in her line of sight. Physically, she was at a risk for falls. Randall identified the following target problems: (1) difficulty engaging Rose in meaningful activities; (2) resistance to bathing and hair washing; and (3) anxiety and yelling out for help.

The couple participated in ten COPE sessions. For each problem, the practitioner implemented the problem-solving and mind-mapping process to identify customized strategies. Probing questions included 'Describe the problem in detail'; 'What exactly bothers you about this problem?'; 'When would you consider this problem solved?'; and 'Where does this problem occur; at what time of day; with whom?' Randall was actively involved in selecting strategies to address each problem that he practised during and in between occupational therapy sessions.

Problem 1: Randall was guided to identify the types of activities that Rose previously enjoyed (including cards, games and organization or household tasks), and was then educated in task simplification strategies to adjust the demand of the activity to meet Rose's capacities. The practitioner helped Randall shift his expectation from Rose doing the activity correctly to focusing on her enjoyment and wellbeing. By 'relaxing the rules' and focusing on sensory-based experiences rather than goal-oriented tasks, Randall was successful in facilitating meaningful engagement with Rose whilst playing an adapted game of cards or sorting coins. Randall learned to adapt his communication style to short phrases in the form of action statements supported by gestures rather than questions: 'Here are the cards!' rather than 'Do you want to play cards?' and 'Great job Rose' instead of 'You made a mistake.' Randall learned to adapt the environment by limiting the number of objects used during a task, as Rose was easily distracted. Setting the activity up in advance allowed Rose to see necessary items (within her direct line of sight). As a result of successfully engaging in meaningful activities, Randall felt great satisfaction and joy, and noted that Rose appeared less anxious.

Problem 2: Through the process of problem-solving, Randall realized Rose was unsure how to get in the shower, which caused her to feel anxious and refuse to get in. The strategies he implemented included modifying the shower to add colour contrast to the floor, so that Rose could be directed where to step, so rather than saying 'Get in the shower', Randall said 'Step onto the red mat.' A handheld shower head and shower chair allowed Rose to sit safely whilst in the shower, as showering was overstimulating. Randall augmented his communication approach by adding encouragement throughout the task to help her stay calm and feel valued. With this technique, Rose successfully had a shower one to two times a week with less anxiety and fear.

Problem 3: During the problem-solving and mind mapping, Randall identified that Rose was most anxious and yelled out when she did not understand what Randall was doing to her (for example, when attempting to brush her teeth or trying to transfer or move her body). Randall learned communication techniques to reduce Rose's fear by building connection prior to touching or presenting items (for example, make eye contact, be in Rose's line of sight, and start with light touch prior to more abrupt movement or contact, such as gently touching her hair or the side of her face prior to presenting the toothbrush). Randall found that by using the strategies of connection prior to providing hands-on care, Rose's oral hygiene went from being a frustrating experience to a pleasant activity.

Conclusion

In adopting TAP and COPE, occupational therapists provide education about the underlying disease processes influencing dementia and aiming to teach caregivers how to take care of themselves. In addition, TAP and COPE support the implementation of strategies that can facilitate activity engagement, reduce behavioural symptoms and promote performance of self-care activities. Critical to both interventions is the focus on generalizing knowledge and skills as the disease progresses. Conceptual models that explain the effect of the physical and social environment on the performance and capacity of the person living with dementia and the readiness of caregivers to implement strategies (that is, change their behaviour) drive the complex nature of clinical reasoning. Collaboration with caregivers is imperative in the process of creating customized strategies that promote effective communication and care approaches, task simplification and environmental modifications. Best practice in dementia care requires educating caregivers at a level that meets their needs, guiding caregivers' implementation of tailored strategies, and promoting their ability to generalize newly learned skills into their daily care routines, including into the future, as the person's function changes.

Reflective questions

1. Why is it imperative to involve caregivers in occupational therapy for people living with dementia?
2. Why do you think active engagement of the caregiver in problem-solving and mind-mapping training is an important part of the COPE intervention?
3. Reflect on a client you have observed living with dementia. Would that client benefit from TAP or COPE, and can you highlight the clinical reasoning influencing your decision?

Acknowledgements

Thank you to Claire Martin, MSc (Pre-Reg) Occupational Therapy, for supporting the writing of the TAP case study.

Caroline Kate Keefe's role was funded in part by grant number 90ADPl006-01-00, from the US Administration for Community Living, Department of Health and Human Services, Washington, DC, 2021. Grantees undertaking projects under government sponsorship are encouraged to express freely their findings and conclusions. Points of view or opinions do not, therefore, necessarily represent official Administration for Community Living policy.

References

Alzheimer Scotland (2012) *Delivering Integrated Dementia Care: The 8 Pillars Model of Community Support*. Edinburgh: Alzheimer Scotland. Accessed on 29/12/2021 at www.alzscot.org/sites/default/files/2019-07/FULL_REPORT_8_Pillars_Model_of_Community_Support.pdf

Alzheimer's Association (2021) *Facts and Figures*. London: Alzheimer's Association. Accessed on 29/12/2021 at www.alz.org/media/Documents/alzheimers-facts-and-figures.pdf

Burch, K.C. and Burch, B.D. (2021) 'Activities of daily living performance in persons with dementia: Comparing care partners' and clinicians' appraisal and associated factors.' *Alzheimer's Disease & Associated Disorders 35*, 2, 153–159.

Fortinsky, R.H., Gitlin, L.N., Pizzi, L.T., Piersol, C.V., *et al.* (2020) 'Effectiveness of the care of persons with dementia in their environments intervention when embedded in a publicly funded home- and community-based service program.' *Innovation in Aging 4*, 6, 1–13. doi:10.1093/geroni/igaa053

Fraker, J., Kales, H.C., Blazek, M., Kavanagh, J. and Gitlin, L.N. (2014) 'The role of the occupational therapist in the management of neuropsychiatric symptoms of dementia in clinical settings.' *Occupational Therapy in Healthcare 28*, 1, 4–20. doi: 10.3109/07380577.2013.867468

Gitlin, L.N., Winter, L., Corcoran, M., Dennis, M., Schinfeld, S. and Hauck, W. (2001) 'A randomized, controlled trial of a home environmental intervention: Effect on efficacy and upset in caregivers and on daily function of persons with dementia.' *The Gerontologist 41*, 4–14.

Gitlin, L.N., Winter, L., Burke, J., Chernett, N., Dennis, M.P. and Hauck, W.W. (2008) 'Tailored activities to manage neuropsychiatric behaviors in persons with dementia: A randomized pilot study.' *American Journal of Geriatric Psychiatry 16*, 3, 229–239. doi:10.1097/JGP.0b013e318160da72

Gitlin, L.N., Winter, L., Earland, T.V., Herge, E.A., *et al.* (2009) 'The tailored activity program (TAP) to reduce behavioral symptoms in individuals with dementia: Feasibility, acceptability, and replication potential.' *The Gerontologist 49*, 428–439. https://doi:10.1093/geront/gnp087

Gitlin, L.N., Jacobs, M. and Earland, T.V. (2010) 'Translation of a dementia caregiver intervention for delivery in homecare as a reimbursable Medicare service: Outcomes and lessons learned.' The Gerontologist 50, 847–854. doi:10.1093/geront/gnq057

Gitlin, L.N., Winter, L., Dennis, M.P., Hodgson, N. and Hauck, W.W. (2010) 'Targeting and managing behavioral symptoms in individuals with dementia: A randomized trial of nonpharmacologic intervention.' Journal of the American Geriatrics Society 58, 8, 1465–1474. doi:10.1111/j.1532-5415.2010.02971.x

Gitlin, L.N. and Rose, K. (2016) 'Impact of caregiver readiness on outcomes of a non-pharmacological intervention to address behavioral symptoms in persons with dementia.' International Journal of Geriatric Psychiatry 6, 31, 1056–1063. doi:10.1002/gps.4422

Gitlin, L.N., Arthur, P., Piersol, C., Dai, Y. and Mann, W.C. (2018) 'Targeting behavioral symptoms and functional decline in dementia: A randomized clinical trial.' Journal of the American Geriatrics Society 66, 339–345. https://doi.org/10.1111/jgs.15194

Lawton, M.P. and Nahemow, L. (1973) 'Ecology and the Aging Process.' In C. Eisdorfer and M.P. Lawton (eds) The Psychology of Adult Development and Aging (pp.619–674). Washington, DC: American Psychological Association. doi:10.1037/10044-020

McCraith, D.B. and Earhart, C.A. (2018) 'Cognitive Disabilities Model: Creating Fit between Functional Cognitive Abilities and Cognitive Activity Demands.' In N. Katz and J. Toglia (eds) Cognition, Occupation, and Participation across the Lifespan (4th edn, pp.469–497). AOTA Press.

Mukherjee, A., Biswas, A., Roy, A., Biswas, S., Gangopadhyay, G. and Das, S.K. (2017) 'Behavioural and psychological symptoms of dementia: Correlates and impact on caregiver distress.' Dementia and Geriatric Cognitive Disorders 7, 354–365. doi:10.1159/000481568

Novelli, M., Machado, S., Lima, G.B., Cantalore, L., et al. (2018) 'Effects of the Tailored Activity Program in Brazil (TAP-BR) for persons with dementia: A randomized pilot trial.' Alzheimer Disease and Associated Disorders 32, 4, 339–345. doi:10.1097/WAD.0000000000000256

Pearlin, L., Menaghan, E., Lieberman, M. and Mullan, J. (1981) 'The stress process.' Journal of Health and Social Behavior 22, 4, 337–356. doi:10.2307/2136676

Piersol, C.V., Herge, E.A., Copolillo, A.E., Leiby, B.E. and Gitlin, L.N. (2016) 'Psychometric properties of the Functional Capacity Card Sort for caregivers of people with dementia.' Occupational Therapy Journal of Research 36, 126–133. doi:10.1177/1539449216666063

Reid, J. (2014) 'Helping People with Dementia to Stay Active in Their Homes.' In Alzheimer Scotland, Allied Health Professionals Delivering Integrated Dementia Care: Living Well with Community Support (pp.16–17). Edinburgh: Alzheimer Scotland. Accessed on 29/12/2021 at www.alzscot.org/sites/default/files/2019-07/AHP_Collaboration%20Document%20-%20Living%20Well%20with%20Community%20Support.pdf

Sivananthan, S.N. and McGrail, K.M. (2016) 'Diagnosis and disruption: Population-level analysis identifying points of care at which transitions are highest for people with dementia and factors that contribute to them.' Journal of the American Geriatrics Society 64, 569–577. doi:10.1111/jgs.14033

WHO (World Health Organization) (2021) 'Dementia.' Fact sheets, 2 September. Accessed on 25/11/2021 at www.who.int/news-room/fact-sheets/detail/dementia

CHAPTER 17

Challenges and Opportunities in Occupational Therapy Intervention Research

Jennifer Wenborn and Alison Warren

> **Learning outcomes**
> By the end of this chapter, you will have the opportunity to:
>
> ▸ Update your knowledge of occupational therapy intervention-related research for people living with dementia and their caregivers
> ▸ Consider the challenges of research methodologies and potential solutions to capture meaningful, occupation-focused change
> ▸ Discover opportunities available to occupational therapists to become involved in research.

Introduction

Research within occupational therapy has gained momentum in making a difference to the lives of people living with dementia and their caregivers. The profession has always believed that its person-centred approach has the potential to promote wellbeing through occupation, and research across the stages of dementia seeks to capture important change. It is an exciting time to be an occupational therapist working in dementia practice, as innovative ways of working with individuals and groups are being researched. This chapter seeks to provide an overview of key occupational therapy intervention research for people living with dementia, identify some challenges and opportunities of research methodologies, and provide practical ideas to encourage occupational therapists and students to engage with research.

As occupational therapists we both became involved in research in our careers due to having enquiring minds and a desire to make a positive difference to the lives of people living with dementia of all ages. Working collaboratively to develop services with an occupation focus led us to identify gaps of knowledge through audits with our occupational therapy colleagues, and highlighted the need to implement research to capture outcomes and develop practice. We have each utilized a range of research methods, and the first author (Jennifer) has extensive experience in designing and conducting randomized controlled trials (RCTs).

We have outstanding occupational therapy researchers leading the way for the profession as well as being key players within interprofessional research teams. Harnessing expertise is key for occupational therapy, and sharing practice ideas and research is essential to highlight the impact we can make on occupational engagement and wellbeing. There have been challenges historically between proving outcomes and capturing change for health conditions that currently have no specific cures. Collaborating with people living with dementia and their caregivers to ensure their expertise by experience is integrated and utilized, taking a co-production approach, throughout the research process is growing.

To capture experiences, change and effectiveness, occupational therapy interventions within dementia care are best thought of as complex interventions. According to the Medical Research Council (MRC) (2008) it can be challenging to identify which elements of complex intervention may be having an effect on a person. The MRC has produced a framework for developing and evaluating complex interventions (MRC 2008), and a guide to process evaluation (Moore *et al.* 2014) that offers valuable guidance on intervention research.

Occupational therapists have incredible skills for enabling individuals with dementia to engage in meaningful occupation, promote or maintain independence as well as supporting caregivers, including family members. Occupational therapy interventions frequently begin with an idea from professional practice, and how this may develop into research often involves exploring individual experiences and qualitative evaluation, to a feasibility study, and then to a pilot trial, and in some areas, an RCT. The challenge is considering where occupational therapists can move their interventions from thinking that something is generating positive change to moving more confidently towards knowing that positive change is possible. It is key to keep this goal in sight.

Involvement in research is core to the development of the profession internationally as well as at an individual level. The World Federation of Occupational Therapists (WFOT) clearly views research as fundamental to developing practice through investigating the effectiveness of occupational therapy interventions and exploring how occupation enables participation in everyday life (WFOT *et al.* 2017). Service user involvement is core to this process, and involving people living with dementia not only as research participants but also through co-production in research is crucial. There are also people living with dementia aiming to develop new approaches through carrying out research that is led and controlled by people with dementia, for example, Dementia Enquirers in the UK (a Dementia Engagement and Empowerment Project (DEEP) project) (Dementia Enquirers n.d.). Working collaboratively with all stakeholders is fundamental to getting useful, focused research to broaden future knowledge. As occupational therapists, through working collaboratively with people living with dementia, research goals can be identified based on what sorts of intervention people want, need and value. Therefore, this chapter seeks to summarize key current research evidence of occupational therapy interventions supporting people living with dementia and their caregivers. It will also provide ideas of how occupational therapists and students can become involved in research to develop interventions, and evaluate and translate evidence-based interventions into practice.

The evidence

This section outlines key evidence supporting the delivery of occupation-focused interventions for people living with dementia. Interventions are not always named as being 'occupational therapy', but occupational therapists have often been involved in the intervention development and delivery within the research study. Therefore, the philosophy of using occupational engagement as either the process and/ or outcome resonates with us as occupational therapists.

The most effective non-pharmacological interventions for people with dementia include a number of related components, such as being tailored to the individual, and educating the caregiver in communication skills and coping strategies (Clarkson *et al.* 2017; Livingston *et al.* 2017, 2020). Hence, many of our interventions are 'dyadic', that is, designed to engage both the person with dementia and their caregiver. In general, these aim to maintain occupational performance and engagement through building on the person with dementia's abilities and skills; helping the caregiver learn communication, supervision and problem-solving strategies; and adapting the environment to maximize engagement. The combination and relative focus of these components varies depending on what stage or severity of dementia the intervention is designed for.

In this section, we outline some key research-based evidence for occupation-focused interventions, starting with those designed for people in the earlier stages. Journeying through Dementia (see Chapter 15) is designed for people in the earlier stages of dementia, having been adapted from the Lifestyle Matters programme (Wright *et al.* 2019). This manualized intervention consists of 12 weekly groups for 8–12 participants, who also have four one-to-one sessions with a facilitator to tackle their individual goals. The aim is to develop skills and techniques that can allow a person living with dementia to continue doing what they enjoy for as long as possible. Participants can involve a supporter, for example, a family member or friend, if they wish. A multisite RCT recruited 480 people with dementia and 350 supporters to test its clinical and cost-effectiveness. The primary quantitative outcome measure initially improved but did not reach statistical significance, meaning that there was no evidence of effectiveness. In contrast, the participants recounted in qualitative interviews very positive accounts of taking part and the intervention's impact.

The community occupational therapy in dementia (COTiD) programme for older people with mild to moderate dementia and their caregivers was developed in the Netherlands (Graff *et al.* 2006). It aimed to improve the person with dementia's activities of daily living (ADL) performance, and their caregiver's supervision and problem-solving skills, thereby increasing the caregiver's sense of competence and decreasing their burden of care. A single-site RCT was conducted with 135 dyads. The person with dementia's ability to perform ADL and the caregiver's sense of competence improved significantly in the intervention group (Graff *et al.* 2006), which was also cost-effective (Graff *et al.* 2008). A multisite German study translated COTiD but found no difference between this and a single occupational therapy consultation visit (Voigt-Radloff *et al.* 2011a). Importantly, the process evaluation highlighted the need to not just translate but also to adapt complex interventions to maximize their relevance and feasibility to other cultures and service contexts before trying to implement and evaluate them (Voigt-Radloff *et al.* 2011b). COTiD is therefore being translated and adapted in other countries.

The Valuing Active Life in Dementia (VALID) research programme translated and adapted COTiD to develop a UK version, COTiD-UK. A multisite RCT (Wenborn *et al.* 2021) recruited 468 dyads. The intervention was delivered with moderate fidelity. There was no statistical evidence supporting the effectiveness of COTiD-UK in any of the outcomes (ADL, quality of life, mood, resource use, caregiver sense of competence). In contrast, the qualitative interviews conducted with the COTiD-UK occupational therapists and dyads reflected a very positive experience. Interviewees valued the occupation focus, the emphasis on working together to enable both the person with dementia and the family member to set and achieve their goals. Dyads reported that they felt better informed and thereby enabled to plan in the short and longer term to live well with dementia (Burgess *et al.* 2020).

Research highlighting the beneficial impact of enabling occupation for care home residents has often not been led by occupational therapists, although it does reflect the reality of working in this sector where we need to promote the message that 'occupation' is everyone's business. Occupational therapists can, of course, act as consultants/educators/supervisors to enable this to happen, but occupational opportunities need to be integrated within daily care provision rather than be delivered according to a rigid timetable of group activities. Wenborn *et al.* (2013) evaluated the effectiveness of an occupational therapist-led programme to train and coach care home staff to increase activity provision to improve quality of life for residents with dementia. This did not provide quantitative evidence for the efficacy of the intervention, although compliance to its delivery varied greatly across the care homes, and so some residents did not actually receive the enhanced activity provision as planned, but the qualitative findings suggested residents who did receive enhanced occupational opportunities had a positive experience.

We are aware that occupational therapists frequently incorporate other evidence-based non-pharmacological interventions into their practice (Livingston *et al.* 2017, 2020), often delivered with an occupational focus. Cognitive stimulation therapy (CST), cognitive rehabilitation and cognitive training are such examples, and we urge readers to check out others, especially those supported by the Cochrane Reviews.

Multisensory interventions, such as rummage bags, sensory cushions and aprons, have been shown to reduce agitation (Livingston *et al.* 2017). A scoping review by Smith and D'Amico (2020) highlighted that sensory-based interventions are being used more frequently with people living with dementia. Animal-assisted therapy (Lai *et al.* 2019) and using dolls and soft toys (Mitchell, McCormack and McCance 2016) can also contribute to a sensory approach. Music can be used as a group or individual intervention, and can include active and/or receptive (or passive) musical elements, for example singing within CST or reminiscence sessions, or alongside care delivery, such as playing personally meaningful music at bathing and mealtimes. Van der Steen *et al.* (2018) found that music-based interventions probably reduce depressive symptoms, improve behavioural problems, and may improve quality of life and reduce anxiety, but may have little effect on cognition.

Ideally all these approaches are informed by knowing the individual's life story, their occupational history, preferences and values, as originally noted by Kitwood (1997). Indeed, life story work can be used an as intervention in its own right (Gridley *et al.* 2016).

Implementing research

The RCT is widely seen as the 'gold standard' research design for demonstrating effectiveness. However, this methodology presents challenges when used to test complex interventions such as occupational therapy (Birken, Wenborn and Connell 2022). Unsurprisingly, the methodology was originally designed for pharmacological, laboratory-based trials, not testing complex interventions in real-life settings, for example in people's homes. Here we consider some of the challenges and opportunities of implementing research methodologies and the need for flexibility and innovation as no 'one size fits all' when designing and conducting studies.

There are ethical considerations to recruiting people with dementia, including the need to assess an individual's mental capacity to make an informed choice about participation and a consultee process for participants who lose capacity during the study. Studies involving dyads increase the complexity of recruitment, as both parties need to consent and participate in the research process, and potentially the intervention – although how do we know if both parties have been involved in the decision-making process? Much depends on the timing and nature of the approach by researchers – it can be perceived as being too early after diagnosis, either because people are still processing the news or they are at the stage where they feel they are managing fine. Also, staff and families can at times make assumptions about a person with dementia's ability or willingness to engage in research studies without even discussing it. This can prevent people making their own decisions and exclude their valuable opinions at various stages of the research process, thus limiting the data collected, as well as being an ethical issue.

An RCT key feature is 'masking' (or 'blinding') the participants' random allocation. We cannot mask participants as to which intervention they have or have not received, and although we can employ strategies to mask those collecting outcome data, risks of unmasking remain. We can remind participants when booking and arriving at follow-up appointments not to mention their allocation, but we are working with people with impaired memory, and so participants may let slip that they had 'enjoyed working with the occupational therapist' or leave intervention materials on display, or the researcher may notice environmental clues such as newly installed assistive technology.

Process evaluation enables us to better understand the intervention implementation, mechanisms of impact and context (Moore *et al.* 2015). It uses quantitative and qualitative methodologies as relevant at each stage. Nested within an RCT it can help us interpret statistical results and consider their generalizability.

Intervention implementation is crucial to consider throughout. First, the intervention must be clearly defined, especially the aim and 'active ingredients'. So how do we 'manualize' a complex person-centred intervention? Qualitative methods at the development, feasibility and piloting stages help us understand the intervention's mechanisms of impact and inform the RCT design and conduct. Interventionists must be trained to deliver the intervention – as defined in the manual and research protocol – and supervised to minimize contamination through introducing other components or intervention 'drift'. Using quantitative methods to assess fidelity of delivery, that is, the extent to which the intervention was delivered as planned within the RCT, enables us to interpret effectiveness data. Whilst we can strive to define and monitor intervention delivery, it is not always possible to do likewise with the comparator intervention that is frequently 'usual care', which invariably differs across and within research sites in a multicentre RCT. 'Mixed methodology' is therefore increasingly used to balance the quantitative and qualitative results, as demonstrated by the studies above that did not achieve statistically significant results but provided strong and positive qualitative data about the experience and impact of the intervention.

Obviously, the choice of outcome measure is key within any RCT. The outcome(s) measured need to reflect the intervention's key aim. This sounds obvious, but we can struggle to find the 'right' measure – and then wonder why the statistical results disappoint us. Maybe the 'perfect' outcome measure does not exist, but avoid tacking portions of measures together. They need to be valid, reliable and sensitive to change for the intended population. It takes time to develop and validate outcome measures, so this may need including in study designs.

In professional practice occupational therapists often use observational assessments that have proven validity, reliability and sensitivity. However, there are resource implications of using occupational therapy-specific measures due to the availability of suitably trained practitioners or researchers, the cost of training and the assessment. There are many measures to choose from, but using such a wide range hinders comparison between studies and meta-analysis that could strengthen our evidence base (Birken *et al.* 2022).

Dementia research has traditionally used outcome measures originally designed for pharmacological trials – usually focused on the level of impairment or deterioration in performing ADL. This does not reflect the positive person-centred and occupational focus of occupational therapy interventions, so we need to develop measures that more realistically measure the occupational outcomes that interventions are designed to achieve. We also need to consider when and how to collect outcome data. At what point do we think the intervention is likely to have most effect?

There has also been a reliance on 'proxy' data, that is, asking the caregiver how they think the person with dementia is functioning or feeling. Asking the person with dementia their own opinion was not seen as feasible or reliable due to issues of recall, but alternative data collection methods are developing to enable the active involvement of people with dementia, including the use of innovative methodologies such as photovoice (Phillipson and Hammond 2018).

How to get involved in research
There are many options and opportunities to explore if you are interested in research throughout your occupational therapy career. For example:

- Become a research participant through responding to requests – this can provide insight into research processes and broaden your research methodology knowledge.
- Join journal clubs, either face-to-face or virtually. These can be profession- or dementia-specific, or cover more varied topics, but all help to develop your knowledge and critical appraisal skills.
- Become involved in audits of dementia service standards to better understand quality processes and identify areas requiring investigation.
- Contact your local Research & Development (R&D) or Research & Innovation (R&I) department to discover if there are studies currently or on the horizon where you could get involved, for example, as an independent rater on trials, facilitating focus groups or being trained as a study interventionist.
- Contribute to a systematic review as a second reviewer. This provides an opportunity to familiarize yourself with the current literature and to increase your confidence in assessing the quality of research.
- Broaden your awareness and knowledge of an evolving range of person-centred, creative and co-production research methodologies that seek to capture the voice and expertise by experience of people with dementia.
- Familiarize yourself with local, national and international research priorities for people living with dementia and the profession of occupational therapy.

Conclusion

Looking to the future, this is a thought-provoking time to be interested in occupational therapy research to support people living with dementia. It is estimated that 40 per cent of dementia worldwide could be prevented or delayed by addressing 12 modifiable risk factors: education, hypertension, hearing impairment, smoking, obesity, depression, physical activity, diabetes, social contact, excessive alcohol consumption, traumatic brain injury and air pollution (Livingston *et al.* 2020; see also Chapter 5 in this book). There are countless opportunities for occupational therapists to use occupation therapeutically and to promote the rights of individuals and communities to enhance their health and wellbeing.

Our profession's holistic approach and occupation focus gives many opportunities for capturing meaningful change as a result of interventions offered. We need to further embrace the co-production of research through creative methods, working together to enhance the voice of people living with dementia and their caregivers. As a profession, occupational therapists are often great collaborators with multiple stakeholders, and can work on teams beyond boundaries for research across all stages of the dementia journey for people of all ages.

It is apparent that occupational therapists are leading and contributing to the growing evidence base of interventions to support people and their families to live well with dementia.

Reflective questions

1. Considering the assessments and outcome measures used in practice, which best capture change in occupational performance, goal-setting or quality of life as a result of an occupational therapy intervention? Why is this?
2. How can co-production be harnessed within the research process?
3. What are the next three steps on your research journey as an occupational therapist to make a positive contribution to people living with dementia and their caregivers?

References

Birken, M., Wenborn, J. and Connell, C. (2022) 'Randomised controlled trials of occupational therapy interventions for people with a mental health condition or dementia: A systematic review of study methods and outcome measurement.' *British Journal of Occupational Therapy*, 1–18. https://doi.org/10.1177/03080226221086206

Burgess, J., Wenborn, J., Di Bona, L., Orrell, M. and Poland, F. (2020) 'Exploring the experiences of taking part in the Community Occupational Therapy in Dementia (COTiD-UK) intervention from the perspective of people with dementia, family carers and occupational therapists.' *Dementia 20*, 6, 2057–2076.

Clarkson, P., Hughes, J., Xie, C., Larbey, M., *et al.* (2017) 'Overview of systematic reviews: Effective home support in dementia care, components and impacts – Stage 1, psychosocial interventions for dementia.' *Journal of Advanced Nursing 73*, 12, 2845–2863.

Dementia Enquirers (no date) Home page. Accessed on 25/10/2021 at https://dementiaenquirers.org.uk

Graff, M.J.L., Vernooij-Dassen, M.J.M., Thijssen, M., Dekker, J., Hoefnagels, W.H.L. and Olde Rikkert, M.G.M. (2006) 'Community based occupational therapy for patients with dementia and their care givers: Randomised controlled trial.' *British Medical Journal 333*, 7580, 1196–1201.

Graff, M.J.L., Adang, E.M.M., Vernooij-Dassen, M.J.M., Dekker, J., *et al.* (2008) 'Community occupational therapy for older patients with dementia and their care givers: Cost effectiveness study.' *British Medical Journal 336*, 7636, 134–138.

Gridley, K., Brooks, J., Birks, Y., Baxter, K. and Parker, G. (2016) 'Improving care for people with dementia: Development and initial feasibility study for evaluation of life story work in dementia care.' *Health Services and Delivery Research 4*, 23.

Kitwood, T. (1997) *Dementia Reconsidered: The Person Comes First*. Buckingham: Open University Press.

Lai, N.M., Chang, S.M.W., Ng, S.S., Tan, S.L., Chaiyakunapruk, N. and Stanaway, F. (2019) 'Animal-assisted therapy for dementia.' *Cochrane Database of Systematic Reviews 11*, Art. No. CD013243.

Livingston, G., Sommerlad, A., Orgeta, V., Costafreda, S.G., *et al.* (2017) 'Dementia prevention, intervention, and care.' *The Lancet 390*, 10113, 2673–2734.

Livingston, G., Huntley, J., Sommerlad, A., Ames, D., *et al.* (2020) 'Dementia prevention, intervention, and care: 2020 report of the Lancet Commission.' *The Lancet 396*, 10248, 413–446.

Mitchell, G., McCormack, B. and McCance, T. (2016) 'Therapeutic use of dolls for people living with dementia: A critical review of the literature.' *Dementia 15*, 5, 976–1001.

Moore, G., Audrey, S., Barker, M., Bond, L., *et al.* (2014) *Process Evaluation of Complex Interventions: Medical Research Council Guidance*. London: Medical Research Council.

MRC (Medical Research Council) (2008) *Developing and Evaluating Complex Interventions: The New Medical Research Council Guidance*. London: MRC.

Phillipson, L. and Hammond, A. (2018) 'More than talking: A scoping review of innovative approaches to qualitative research involving people with dementia.' *International Journal of Qualitative Methods 17*, 1, 1–17.

Smith, B.C. and D'Amico, M. (2020) 'Sensory-based interventions for adults with dementia and Alzheimer's disease: A scoping review.' *Occupational Therapy in Health Care 34*, 3, 171–201.

van der Steen, J.T., Smaling, H.J.A., van der Wouden, J.C., Bruinsma, M.S., *et al.* (2018) 'Music-based therapeutic interventions for people with dementia.' *Cochrane Database of Systematic Reviews 7*, Art. No. CD003477.

Voigt-Radloff, S., Graff, M., Leonhart, R., Schornstein, K., *et al.* (2011a) 'A multicentre RCT on community occupational therapy in Alzheimer's disease: 10 sessions are not better than one consultation.' *BMJ Open 1*, 1, e000096.

Voigt-Radloff, S., Graff, M., Leonhart, R., Hüll, M., *et al.* (2011b) 'Why did an effective Dutch complex psycho-social intervention for people with dementia not work in the German healthcare context? Lessons learnt from a process evaluation alongside a multicentre RCT.' *BMJ Open 1*, 1, e000094.

Wenborn, J., Challis, D., Head, J., Miranda-Castillo, C., *et al.* (2013) 'Providing activity for people with dementia in care homes: A cluster randomised controlled trial.' *International Journal of Geriatric Psychiatry 28*, 12, 1296–1304. doi:10.1002/gps.3960

Wenborn, J., O'Keeffe, A.G., Mountain, G., Moniz-Cook, E., *et al.* (2021) 'Community Occupational Therapy for people with dementia and family carers (COTiD-UK) versus treatment as usual (Valuing Active Life in Dementia [VALID] study): A single-blind, randomised controlled trial.' *Trials 17*, 65. doi:10.1186/s13063-015-1150-y

WFOT (World Federation of Occupational Therapists), Mackenzie, L., Coppola, S., Alvarez, L., *et al.* (2017) 'International occupational therapy research priorities.' *OTJR: Occupation, Participation and Health 37*, 2, 72–81.

Wright, J., Foster, A., Cooper, C., Sprange, K., *et al.* (2019) 'Study protocol for a randomised controlled trial assessing the clinical and cost-effectiveness of the Journeying through Dementia (JtD) intervention compared to usual care.' *BMJ Open 9*, e029207. doi:10.1136/bmjopen-2019-029207

Epilogue

Fiona Maclean, Elaine Hunter, Lyn Westcott and Alison Warren

In coming to a close, this Epilogue presents an opportunity to reflect on the initial conversations we had as editors, which led to this publication. In looking back there was a clear commitment from all of us that we wanted to join the wider discourse about the potential contribution of a rights-based approach to occupational therapy dementia practice, and in so doing, to aspire to evolve these conversations, and to further progress professional contribution when working with people living with dementia, their families and caregivers. Consequently, in this final chapter, we briefly revisit our reasons for wanting to contribute to this debate, consider where this leaves us with respect to the content presented in this book, and finally, present our hopes for the future.

Joining a conversation

In choosing to join a conversation about the need to promote and consider what a rights-based approach to occupational therapy dementia practice may look like, one reason was key. The contribution of occupational therapy is increasingly understood to be a central component of the way(s) in which people living with dementia can continue to live positive lives for longer. Moreover, that crucial to person-centred, rights-based occupational therapy dementia practice is an appreciation of 'what you do is you'. The profession prizes participation in occupations that can promote health and wellbeing, which, in turn, characterize who we are and represent the essence and heartbeat of what makes our lives worth living.

A diagnosis of dementia should not alter this certainty. That to sustain and maintain the rhythm of our 'everyday' – everyday occupations identified by people living with dementia as important to them – is not only occupationally just, but represents a human right. Yet, as many of the chapters have indicated here, all too often the occupational possibilities of those living with dementia can be overlooked – the right to sustain a personal life ignored; abilities, rather than disability, disregarded.

As editors of this book, we came together in a spirit of response. For some of us, we have been touched by dementia in both our personal and professional lives, and this undoubtedly influenced why we were drawn to edit this particular publication. However, more importantly, we wanted to make a constructive contribution to the lives of people living with dementia, their families and caregivers. We have therefore worked to bring people, and their expertise, together, to offer an opportunity for students and graduates of occupational therapy to engage with and absorb the nature, scope and potential of their dementia practice.

Ever-evolving conversations

On reading this book, we hope you will have been inspired by our contributors and have had the opportunity to reflect on the questions posed at the end of each chapter. In the text we have shared current practice, research and narratives in dementia, inviting you to keep the conversation going, and to continue to critically reflect on and develop your own practice when working with a person with dementia, their families and caregivers. The generosity of all our authors of their time and commitment to share their thinking in no more than 4000 words in each chapter has been awe-inspiring to us as editors. However, this is not the end of the narrative on occupational therapy and dementia; indeed, we hope it will just be the beginning, as there is so much more. Whilst we have offered a moment in time to a range of occupational therapy interventions, research and debates, as an editing team, we did not have enough pages to share all the work we know will be happening globally. For example:

- *Rights:* We need to consider the rights of people with dementia who are not yet diagnosed, and this may be as high as 90 per cent in some low- and middle-income countries, where stigma and lack of awareness of dementia remain major barriers to diagnosis (Alzheimer's Society 2021). Going forward as a profession, we need to consider, for example, the anecdotal evidence from projects that tell us that LGBT people living with dementia face particular challenges when accessing dementia care services and housing providers (LGBT Foundation 2017).

- *Opportunities:* We need to evolve the opportunities that new research will offer, in areas of therapeutic interventions, brain health, technology and medicine, including how this might influence and enhance existing person-centred rights-based practice, whilst also measuring impact.
- *Reflections:* We still need to reflect on the role of occupational therapy for people with learning disabilities, particularly those with Down's syndrome, who we know are at increased risk of developing dementia (Alzheimer's Society 2021). We also already know people from minority ethnic backgrounds might be more likely to develop dementia than the white British population (NIHR 2021), and thus our research and practice must be representative and reflect the needs of entire communities.

People with dementia are also shaping how we understand their lived experience, challenging us to be bold in our role as occupational therapists, to promote the right to rehabilitation, including the development of seamless pathways of support that include access to occupational therapy, provided for all people living with dementia. Consequently, in looking ahead, we suggest adopting rights, opportunities, and reflections (or ROAR) as a framework through which occupational therapists can share ideas presented in this textbook. To use the acronym of ROAR to shape how and in what way you can contribute to the lives of people living with dementia by recognizing that:

R is for *Rights*, to respect and advocate for the rights of people living with dementia, regardless of where you practice as an occupational therapist.

O is for *Opportunities*, to encourage you to seize every opportunity to make a positive difference when working with people living with dementia, their families and caregivers.

AND

R is for *Reflections*, to encourage you to take time to integrate and critically consider the reflective questions we have posed throughout this book, as part of your future practice.

We would like to invite you to embrace the ROAR acronym, and to always be proud of your work in occupational therapy and dementia.

Continuing the conversation

This book is coming to an end, and it is a good time to consider what you may have learned from your engagement with the writing included here. These chapters, framed by the themes of 'person', 'environment' and 'occupation', (we hope) have stimulated you to think about the ways occupational therapists work alongside people living with dementia, their families and their caregivers. We have provided you, our reader, with opportunities to reflect and interact with what the contributors have thought and said. Hopefully you have had your views about occupational therapy and dementia developed, affirmed or challenged by engaging with the text. If your experience has done one or more of these things, then as editors we feel the book has achieved what we hoped. We have included a wide range of contributors: people living with dementia, people living alongside people with dementia or working with people who live with dementia. Indeed, the writing process has been extremely collegiate throughout, and has brought our contributors together, strengthening our shared purpose.

The writings and conversations presented here are designed to continue looking forwards, gathering momentum and stimulating further critical reflection and actions, actions that can continue to lead, advance and progress occupational therapy dementia research, policy and practice. Like all good conversations, we hope you will feel curious to continue this process, that you will leave this book wanting to find out more, do more and inspire others to become involved in this exciting area for occupational therapists. We thank you for engaging with us in this book, and wish you well in your future conversations, which should always include the voices of people living with dementia.

No matter what the diagnosis is, always make sure you see the person as a person. (Margaret, SDWG member)

References

Alzheimer's Society (2021) *Learning Disabilities and Dementia*. London: Alzheimer's Society. Accessed on 06/12/21 at www.alzheimers.org.uk/about-dementia/types-dementia/learning-disabilities-dementia

LGBT Foundation (2017) *Bring Dementia Out*. Manchester: LGBT Foundation. Accessed on 06/12/21 at https://lgbt.foundation/bringdementiaout

NIHR (National Institute for Health and Care Research) (2020) 'People with dementia from ethnic minority backgrounds face extra barriers in accessing care.' Brain and Nerves, 4 December. Accessed on 06/12/21 at https://evidence.nihr.ac.uk/alert/ethnic-minority-dementia-extra-barriers-in-accessing-care

About the Authors

Anna Borthwick, Executive Lead at Brain Health Scotland, Alzheimer Scotland, Edinburgh, UK.

Dr Hannah Bradwell, Digital Health Research Fellow, University of Plymouth, England, UK.

Dr Margaret Brown, Senior Lecturer and Deputy Director, Alzheimer Scotland Centre for Policy and Practice, University of the West of Scotland, South Lanarkshire, Scotland, UK.

Dr Kari Burch, Occupational Therapist, Memory Care Home Solutions, St Louis, Missouri, USA.

Jill Cigliana, Program Director, Memory Care Home Solutions, St Louis, Missouri, USA.

Liz Copley, Consultant Occupational Therapist, Older People's Mental Health, Rotherham, Doncaster and South Humber NHS Foundation Trust, England, UK.

Professor Claire Craig, Professor of Design and Creative Practice in Health and Co-Director, Lab4Living, Sheffield Hallam University, England, UK.

Kimberley Crocker-White, Occupational Therapist in a Dementia and Older People's Mental Health Service, Cornwall Partnership NHS Foundation Trust, England, UK.

Sophia Dickinson, Occupational Therapy Consultant, Director, Home Independence Occupational Therapy Ltd, Leicester, England, UK.

Katie Edwards, Research Associate in Digital Health, University of Plymouth, England, UK.

Dr Michelle Elliot, Senior Lecturer, Division of Occupational Therapy and Arts Therapies, Queen Margaret University, Edinburgh, Scotland, UK.

Helen Fisher, Research Associate, Department of Art and Design, working with Lab4Living, Sheffield Hallam University, England, UK.

Fiona Fraser, Programme Lead and Lecturer in Occupational Therapy, University of Plymouth, England, UK.

Neil Fullerton, Project and Communications Lead at Brain Health Scotland, Alzheimer Scotland, Edinburgh, UK.

Jayne Goodrick, Dementia Activists, expert by experience, carer for person with dementia, Volunteer, Wales, UK.

Gill Gowran, Advanced Practitioner Occupational Therapist, NHS Lanarkshire, Scotland, UK.

Ashleigh Gray, Occupational Therapist, Older Adult Community Mental Health Team, NHS Fife, Scotland, UK.

Angela Gregory, PhD student, HCPC-registered Occupational Therapist, University of the West of Scotland, UK.

Dr Clare Hocking, Professor of Occupational Science and Therapy, Auckland University of Technology, New Zealand.

Elaine Hunter, National Allied Health Professions Consultant, Alzheimer Scotland, and Visiting Professor, Edinburgh Napier University, Edinburgh, UK.

Dr Sarah Kantartzis, Senior Lecturer, Queen Margaret University, Edinburgh, UK.

Caroline Kate Keefe, OTD, OTR/L, Therapy Practice Lead, LiveWell Dementia Specialists, Plantsville, Connecticut, USA.

Dr Debbie Laliberte Rudman, Distinguished University Professor, School of Occupational Therapy, University of Western Ontario, Canada.

Dr Fiona Maclean, Associate Professor of Occupational Therapy, Edinburgh Napier University, UK.

Margaret McCallion, SDWG member, Alzheimer Scotland, UK.

Professor Brendan McCormack, Head of School and Dean, Susan Wakil School of Nursing and Midwifery, Sydney Nursing School Faculty of Medicine and Health, and President Omega Xi Chapter Sigma Global.

Mary McGrath, Principal Occupational Therapist, Belfast Health and Social Care Trust, Northern Ireland, UK.

Professor Elizabeth Anne McKay, Lead Allied Health Professions & Social Work, Edinburgh Napier University, Scotland, UK.

Alison McKean, Allied Health Professional Post Diagnostic Lead, Alzheimer Scotland, UK.

Lorna Noble, SDWG member, Alzheimer Scotland, UK.

Dr Maria O'Reilly, Head of Course – Occupational Therapy, School of Health, Medical and Applied Sciences, Central Queensland University, Bundaberg, Australia.

Dr Toni M. Page, Digital Health Research Fellow, Centre for Health Technology, University of Plymouth, England, UK.

Dr Catherine Verrier Piersol, Professor and Chair, Department of Occupational Therapy, Thomas Jefferson University, Philadelphia, Pennsylvania, USA.

Jackie Pool, Dementia Care Champion, Quality Compliance Systems Ltd, Uxbridge, England, UK.

Henry Rankin, SDWG member, Alzheimer Scotland, UK.

Wendy Rankin, Active Voice Lead, SDWG, Alzheimer Scotland, UK.

Chris Roberts, Dementia Activists, expert by experience living with dementia, Volunteer, Wales, UK.

Lynsey Robertson, Occupational Therapist, NHS Scotland, UK.

Dr Anthony Schrag, Senior Lecturer in Arts Management and Cultural Policy, Queen Margaret University, Edinburgh, Scotland, UK.

Ian Kenneth Grant Sherriff BEM, Academic Partnership Lead for Dementia, Faculty of Medicine, Dentistry and Allied Health, University of Plymouth, England, UK.

Dr Katherine Turner, Lecturer in Occupational Therapy, School of Health Professions, University of Plymouth, England, UK.

Dr Alison Warren, Associate Professor of Occupational Therapy, School of Health Professions, University of Plymouth, England, UK.

Dr Jennifer Wenborn, Honorary Senior Clinical Research Fellow and Occupational Therapist, Division of Psychiatry, University College London, England, UK.

Lyn Westcott, Professional Lead and Consultant in Occupational Therapy, University of Hertfordshire, Hatfield, England, UK.

Subject Index

Author Index